Safeguarding and Child Protection for Nurses, Midwives and Health Visitors

Safeguarding and Child Protection for Nurses, Midwives and Health Visitors

A Practical Guide

Second Edition

Catherine Powell

Open University Press

Open University Press
McGraw-Hill Education
McGraw-Hill House
Shoppenhangers Road
Maidenhead
Berkshire
England
SL6 2QL

email: enquiries@openup.co.uk
world wide web: www.openup.co.uk

and Two Penn Plaza, New York, NY 10121-2289, USA

First published 2011
First published in this second edition 2016

A catalogue record of this book is available from the British Library

ISBN-13: 978-0-33-526252-6
ISBN-10: 0-33-526252-X
eISBN: 978-0-33-526253-3

Library of Congress Cataloging-in-Publication Data
CIP data applied for

Typeset by SPi-Global

Printed and bound by CPI Group (UK) Ltd, Croydon, CR0 4YY

Praise for this book

"*Dr Catherine Powell is the Institute of Health Visiting safeguarding expert, advising us on any national safeguarding issues or changes of policy. I am personally delighted that she has updated this important book. Safeguarding is the practice area that nurses, midwives and health visitors must not shy away from. It can however provide their greatest professional challenges as well as making them feel anxious about providing correct professional responses.*

This is a very well-structured and comprehensive book. The author very effectively brings safeguarding responsibilities to life with the use of case studies. The recurring features in the book are helpful and I very much like the inclusion of the child or young person's perspective boxes. For the inexperienced professional this can be forgotten when swamped with a complex situation. By keeping the child's perspective at the centre of all decision-making the right decisions are more likely to be made.

Perhaps of particular value to learning will be the chapter on child death and serious case reviews, something professionals seek to avoid ever being involved in, but sometimes find themselves having to face. It is therefore important to learn from these reviews of what went wrong, a breakdown in professional communication so often being a feature. This chapter explains how a serious case review is carried out and allows the reader to understand how they might be asked to contribute to the process.

To have a book such as this to use as a professional companion, not only to refer to and check facts, or underpin decision making, but also to expand professional knowledge, will lead to improved safeguarding practices, prompt, appropriate interventions, and better outcomes for children and families. Safeguarding is of course everyone's business and others needing to refresh or update their skills in this area will also find the information included of great value."

Dr Cheryll Adams, Director, Institute of Health Visiting, UK

"*This is a very readable and practical book which achieves its aim to raise awareness about good safeguarding and child protection practice. The book is intended to prepare nursing, midwifery and specialist community public health nursing students and those 'returning to practice', but it will also be of use to more experienced practitioners who work with children, young people and their families, wanting to update their learning in the field.*

The book clearly reflects the author's expertise and knowledge in safe-guarding and child protection practice. It contains a wealth of extremely useful information presented in an easily accessible fashion. The range of case examples, practice points and new for this second edition, a 'child's perspective' box, brings the text to life and focuses the reader's attention on practice needing to be 'child-centred'. This is an excellent book, which I thoroughly recommend."

Jane V. Appleton, Professor in Primary and Community Care, Faculty of Health and Life Sciences at Oxford Brookes University, UK

"All nurses have a duty to inform and alert appropriate personnel if they suspect a child has been abused, and to know where they can seek expert advice and support if they have concerns. This comprehensive text provid-ing the link between legislation, policy, research and practice will enable students and practitioners to expand their knowledge and understanding of the key issues involved in safeguarding children and young people."

Fiona Smith, Professional Lead for Children and Young People's Nursing, Royal College of Nursing, UK

For the professionals who improve the lives of children, young people and their families – with thanks

Contents

About the Author

Catherine Powell is a Safeguarding Children Consultant and Visiting Academic at the University of Southampton, UK.

Abbreviations

ACE	adverse events in childhood
ADHD	attention deficit hyperactive disorder
CAF	Common Assessment Framework
CAMHS	child and adolescent mental health services
CASH	contraception and sexual health
CBT	cognitive behavioural therapy
CCG	clinical commissioning group
CDOP	child death overview panel
CEOP	Child Exploitation and Online Protection Centre
CQC	Care Quality Commission
CSE	child sexual exploitation
CT	computerized tomography
DKA	diabetic ketoacidosis
DOSC	designated officer for safeguarding children
DVA	domestic violence and abuse
ED	emergency department
EHA	Early Help Assessment
EHC	education and health care plan
FGM	female genital mutilation
FII	fabricated or induced illness
FNP	Family Nurse Partnership
GIRFEC	Getting it Right for Every Child
GP	general practitioner
ICPC	initial child protection conference
LADO	local authority designated officer
LSCB	Local Safeguarding Children Board
MAPPA	multi-agency public protection arrangements
MARAC	multi-agency risk assessment conferencing
MASH	multi-agency safeguarding hub

NEET	not in education, employment or training
NICE	National Institute for Health and Clinical Excellence
NMC	Nursing and Midwifery Council
NSPCC	National Society for the Prevention of Cruelty to Children
ODD	oppositional defiant disorder
Ofsted	Office for Standards in Education, Children's Services and Skills
PEG	percutaneous endoscopic gastrostomy
PICU	paediatric intensive care unit
PSHE	personal, social and health education
RAD	reflex anal dilation
RCPC	review child protection conference
SARC	sexual assault and referral centre
SCR	serious case review
SENCO	special educational needs coordinator
SERAF	Sexual Exploitation Risk Assessment Framework (tool)
SIDS	sudden infant death syndrome
SIRI	serious incident requiring investigation
SUDI	sudden unexpected death in infancy
TAC	team around the child
TAF	team around the family
TPKE	Teenage Pregnancy Knowledge Exchange
UNCRC	United Nations Convention on the Rights of the Child 1989
WHO	World Health Organization
WNB	was not brought

Introduction to the second edition

I am delighted to have been given the opportunity by Open University Press to produce a second edition of this practical guide on safeguarding and child protection for nurses, midwives and health visitors. I am humbled by the feedback that I have received regarding the apparent usefulness of first edition, and hope that this updated text will equally generate both greater confidence in, and wider acknowledgement of, the vital role of nursing, midwifery and health visiting in the prevention, recognition and response to children and young people who are at risk of, or suffering from, child maltreatment.

The book was conceived in recognition that we belong to a large and potent workforce with a range of opportunities to make a difference. Our strength is that we bridge universal and specialist services in maternity, child health, mental health, learning disabilities and adult health. Our practice takes place in a wide range of settings with the health of children, young people and their families being at the heart of what we do. We also understand that there are a broad range of behaviours in the way in which families function and the way in which children are parented and cared for. Because of this, we are in an excellent position to spot situations that may fall outside of the norm and pose a threat to the safety and the well-being of the most vulnerable individuals in our care.

Safeguarding is a core professional responsibility. However, if you are a nursing, midwifery or specialist community public health nursing student[1] or a newly qualified practitioner, the chances are that you may be feeling anxious about 'getting it right'. You may also feel overwhelmed by the vast array of local and national policies and procedures that provide the framework for safeguarding and child protection practice. The over-arching purpose of this practical text is thus to develop your knowledge, skills and competence so that you can help to ensure that the potential of the professions' contribution to ensuring the safety and well-being of children and young people is realized.

This book is primarily aimed at nursing, midwifery and health visiting students and newly qualified professionals, who will ultimately be accountable for their safeguarding and child protection practice. However, it is likely that there will be more experienced practitioners, perhaps those working

[1]The specialist community public health nurse part of the NMC Register includes health visitors and school nurses.

essentially with adult groups, who have had little opportunity to develop their knowledge, skills and competence in safeguarding and child protection practice. These practitioners may find that this book offers new perspectives on their role and the statutory expectations placed on them to recognize and respond to concerns about a child or young person. Another important group of professionals will be those 'returning to practice' after a gap in their nursing, midwifery or health visiting careers. These 'returners' may find that their safeguarding and child protection knowledge is a little rusty, and will find that this book ensures an accessible means to revisit it and to update. In addition, there will be those from outside the nursing and midwifery professions who would benefit from a greater understanding of the potential safeguarding contribution of these professionals. These may include staff in partner agencies and those taking up new commissioning responsibilities for groups of health care professionals (as is the case for local authorities in England). In short, this practical text may appeal to a wider audience than is initially evident.

Promoting the welfare of children and young people, and ensuring that they are protected from harm is, in my view, one of the most challenging, yet also rewarding, aspects of professional practice. Safeguarding and child protection work cuts across 'branches', 'sub-disciplines', 'specialties' and 'settings'. It places nurses, midwives and health visitors as valued partners within the context of multi-professional and inter-agency working; especially in partnership with colleagues from children's social care, the police and education. Safeguarding children is a key public health and it is a whole-profession responsibility.

Media representation of the professional contribution to safeguarding and child protection can give an unfair picture of the reality in practice. It is reasonable to suggest that good safeguarding and child protection practice across all agencies remains largely hidden and unannounced; after all, it is difficult to capture evidence of successfully *preventing* harm. However, anyone whose work brings them into contact with families may come across situations that present a significant risk to children and young people, where children are being harmed and (rarely) the serious injury or death of a child from maltreatment (abuse and neglect). Reviews of such cases offer insights into good practice, as well as opportunities for learning and improvement.

This book, as with the first edition, recognizes that safeguarding and child protection is fundamentally a public health issue, with a public health solution. This means that the contents have been structured in a way that ensures that the public health contribution of the nursing, midwifery and health visiting professions is recognized. The text thus encompasses a wide range of professional activities, including:

- preventative work;
- holistic assessment;
- identification of need;
- provision of 'early help';

- support for parents, and for parenting;
- recognition and referral of children who are at risk of, or are suffering from, significant harm;
- working with a multi-agency team to provide additional support and monitoring as part of a 'child in need' plan or a 'child protection plan'; and
- learning from child death and serious case reviews.

Importantly, a key message for the nursing and midwifery professions is that the skills needed to achieve good safeguarding and child protection practice are very similar to the skills needed to be a good nurse, midwife or health visitor. As I argued in a previous book, nursing and midwifery share some of the core attributes of successful safeguarding practice, including: 'assessing need, working in partnership with individual children and young people, their families and multi-disciplinary teams to promote physical and emotional well-being and ensure safety' (Powell 2007:15–16).

Practice is at the heart of this book. In my own practice I see many examples of the challenging and emotionally demanding work that nurses, midwives and health visitors undertake at the front line to ensure that families are supported, and that children and young people are safe and healthy. These unsung achievements are often remarkable, but there is always more to do. In the words of the late Tony Morrison (2009), my aim as a safeguarding lead has always been to act as a 'scholar-facilitator' – promoting excellence in evidence-informed practice. In doing so, I find that the best learning comes from reflecting on the reality of practice and the *stories* of the families and professionals involved. This book is thus based on case scenarios in practice. These are, for obvious reasons, fictitious and/or anonymized cases, but the events described are all based on reality; the experiences of children, young people, families and professionals who I have been privileged to meet over many years in practice and from whom we can all learn so much.

If you are familiar with the first edition of this book, then you may be interested to know at the outset what has changed in this new extended edition. The most obvious updates are those reflecting NHS structural changes in England, the new Nursing and Midwifery Council (NMC) code and changes to safeguarding and child protection policy within the four countries of the UK. I have also revisited the evidence base for practice, bringing in new resources and ensuring that web-based references remain valid and accessible. There is a new chapter, Chapter 6, which enables more comprehensive coverage of child sexual exploitation (CSE), a topic that has become the focus of public, professional and political attention over the past few years. Drawing on the learning from some of the high-profile cases that have been portrayed in the media, the chapter discusses the challenges of recognition and response to this pernicious form of maltreatment. Additional material has been added throughout to ensure that the book continues to reflect contemporary practice and supports a skilled response to children, young people and families of concern.

As with the first edition, each chapter contains 'practice points', 'practice questions' and 'markers of good practice' to stimulate further thinking and application to real-life practice. New for the second edition is the addition of a recurring 'child's perspective' box that aims to encourage practitioners to actively consider what life is like for the child (Laming 2009) and to support a notion of practice needing to be truly child centred.

Each chapter also begins with a set of 'learning outcomes' and ends with a 'summary' and 'key points' to support practitioner learning.

The first chapter considers the *underpinning principles and frameworks* for safeguarding and child protection practice. This includes a brief overview of contemporary policy and the professional mandate for this work. While the book concerns the safeguarding and child protection work of nurses, midwives and health visitors, this chapter also introduces the roles of others, including the statutory lead agencies (children's social care and the police).

Chapter 2 considers the roles of nurses and midwives in *prevention and early help* and reflects the importance of ensuring the right support and help for children, young people and families with additional needs. The three case scenarios discuss a pregnant 16-year-old, who is referred to the family nurse partnership, a family struggling to cope with the demands of parenting two small boys and a young teenager who is under pressure from her boyfriend to have a sexual relationship. A midwife, a health visitor and a school nurse feature.

Chapter 3 considers *physical abuse* and the process of referral of a child protection concern to children's social care, and introduces the 'strategy discussion'. The three case scenarios discuss a 10-week-old baby who presents with a bruise, a 14-month-old child with suspicious burns and a 6-year-old who is presenting with possible fabricated illness. A practice nurse, an emergency nurse practitioner and a paediatric nurse are key care providers.

Chapter 4 considers *emotional abuse* and the process of the initial child protection conference. The three case scenarios discuss a 6-year-old child described by her mother as 'difficult to love', a 13-year-old who is missing school because she is caring for her younger siblings and a 9-year-old child with cerebral palsy who is somewhat excluded from family life. The children and their families receive care from a child and adolescent mental health practitioner, a school nurse and a community children's nurse.

Chapter 5 considers *sexual abuse* and the professional contribution to a child protection plan. The three case scenarios discuss a 14-year-old attending a young person's sexual health clinic, a 10-year-old with a progressive neurological disorder and an adult mental health client who discloses accessing child pornography on the internet. Care is provided by a sexual health nurse, a learning disability nurse and an adult mental health nurse.

Chapter 6 considers *child sexual exploitation* as a form of child sexual abuse. The three case scenarios discuss a 16-year-old who has presented to the emergency department for the fourth time, a 14-year-old presenting at a contraception and sexual health service for a second termination and a 15-year-old looked-after child, who is having a health review. Practitioners involved in the cases include a triage nurse, a young person's sexual health nurse and a looked-after children's nurse.

Chapter 7 considers *neglect* and the decision-making process at a child protection review conference. The three case scenarios discuss a newborn baby at risk of neglect because of his mother's lifestyle, 18-month-old twins who have been subject to a child protection plan because of concerns about their health and development and a 4-year-old who was admitted to a paediatric intensive care unit after accidentally ingesting an opiate substitute. Practitioners involved in the cases include a midwife, a health visitor and a substance misuse worker.

Chapter 8 considers statutory *serious case review* and *child death review* processes. The cases discussed reflect the death of a teenager in the context of neglect of a health care condition and the sudden unexpected death of an infant. Nurses, midwives and health visitors may be asked to contribute to child death and serious case review processes, albeit that they will be led and supported by safeguarding children specialists. The role of named and designated nurses in these processes is briefly described.

The final chapter, Chapter 9, pulls together the *key learning* with some messages for the future. The Appendix provides an overview of, and reference to, the safeguarding and child protection policy for each of the countries that make up the UK: England, Wales, Scotland and Northern Ireland.

Whether you are a student, a newly qualified practitioner, an experienced practitioner who is seeking to improve her safeguarding children knowledge and skills, you are returning to practice or you have an interest in the potential of the contribution of the nursing and midwifery professions, I hope that you will also find this new edition helpful. Your contribution to keeping children and young people safe is vital; as is your ability to provide help and support to parents, and to support good parenting. You are a highly skilled professional who will have a range of to make a difference; you may even save a life.

1
Principles for practice

Learning outcomes

This chapter will help you to:

- Define key terms – i.e. child, childhood, parenting, safeguarding, child protection and child maltreatment.
- Understand why the needs of the child or young person take priority in decision-making in practice.
- Recognize your statutory and professional duty to safeguard and promote the welfare of children within a context of inter-agency working.
- Map safeguarding and child protection practice to a public health model that promotes prevention.
- Use the remaining chapters to build and inform your knowledge, skills and competence in safeguarding children practice.

Introduction

Prompt recognition to ensure the protection of individuals who are vulnerable or at risk is a core aspect of the code of professional standards of practice and behaviour for nurses and midwives (NMC 2015). The aim of this book is to prepare and support health practitioners to achieve excellence in safeguarding and child protection in their professional role. The book is intended for nursing, midwifery and specialist community public health nursing students, qualified practitioners, those 'returning to practice' and those with an interest in the professional contribution of this workforce within the UK. Above all, it is about supporting best outcomes for children and young people; especially in ensuring their health, safety and well-being.

This opening chapter outlines the principles for safeguarding children practice and provides the foundation for an understanding of the content and context of this book. Key terms are defined, and the legislation and statutory frameworks for developing and supporting professional practice are introduced, as are the roles of other key players in the field. The aim of the chapter is to 'set the scene' for the case studies and practice scenarios that will show how nurses, midwives and health visitors can, and do, play a major role in safeguarding and child protection. This is achieved through a brief review of the underpinning knowledge and skills for practice.

Children and young people

The UK has adopted the legal definition of a child as being an individual who has not yet reached the age of 18 years. This is in line with the United Nations Convention on the Rights of the Child 1989 (hereafter referred to as the UNCRC) and is the definition used within the UK's safeguarding guidance, policy and legislation. The definition applies to all children and young people, including those who are living independently, in further education, the armed forces, or in custody in the secure estate. The fact that childhood includes individuals up to the age of 18 years is important to note, not least because health care traditions in the UK means that those aged 16 and 17 years are likely to be cared for by adult services and in adult settings.[1] In these circumstances, young people will inevitably receive their nursing care and medical treatment from professionals whose preparation for practice has been focused on 'adults'. Such practitioners are likely to be less well briefed, or focused, on their safeguarding and child protection responsibilities.

It is also important to consider the other 'end' of the age spectrum – i.e. the unborn infant. While unborn infants (of any gestation) are not legally defined as children, their need for protection from harm must still be considered in cases where there is concern about expectant parents' ability to ensure the safety and well-being of their child. This would primarily be the responsibility of the midwife and other professionals providing care in the antenatal period. However, because such concerns can relate to substance misuse and/or adult mental health problems or learning disabilities, practitioners working in these fields also need to be aware of their responsibilities to recognize and respond to the risks to the unborn child. It is also pertinent to note that in some cases the 'parent to be' may be a child themselves.

Childhood is clearly a time of rapid, if sometimes uneven, maturity in a multi-faceted range of attributes, including those relating to physical, psychological, intellectual, emotional and social development. Nevertheless, despite the fact that the term 'child' legally applies up until the age of 18 years, this label may not be well received by those developmentally maturing individuals approaching the end of their childhood! Clinical guidelines on child maltreatment commissioned by the National Institute for Health and Clinical Excellence (NICE) (often referred to as the 'NICE guidelines') offer the definitions outlined below and these definitions will be broadly reflected within this book:

- Infant: aged under 1 year
- Child: aged under 13 years
- Young person: aged 13–17 years

(NCCWCH 2009:1)

---

[1] Child and adolescent mental health services (CAMHS) being an important exception.

Practice question

What do you think are the particular care and development needs of individuals within each of the above age groups throughout their journey into adulthood?

Children's rights

The issue of children's rights is an important facet of safeguarding and child protection practice. Nurses, midwives and health visitors may be in a position where they act as an advocate for a child to ensure that their needs are recognized and that they are helped accordingly. Children and young people's rights to provision for welfare and protection from harm, detailed within the UNCRC, are a useful starting point for developing an understanding of what needs to happen in practice to ensure that actions are taken to safeguard and promote their welfare. The UNCRC outlines the responsibilities of governments to provide the best possible services to support children to achieve their full potential into adulthood – i.e. through health, education and social care provision. It also puts in place an expectation that member states will seek to address inequalities between children and adults (e.g. equal right to physical integrity; meaning that children and young people should not be subject to physical punishment, such as being hit).

The UNCRC has four core principles:

- non-discrimination;
- devotion to the best interests of the child;
- the right to life, survival and development;
- respect for the views of the child.

Crucially, the document provides a mandate for the development of a rights-based approach to safeguarding and child protection policy, legislation and guidance, and this is reflected in the UK and Ireland. International readers will need to find out how their governments have enshrined the principles of the UNCRC within their own country's safeguarding and child protection framework.

Importantly, the UNCRC seeks to ensure that children are seen *and* heard. In his report into progress made in safeguarding and child protection in England post the Victoria Climbié tragedy, Laming (2009) argues that the child's perspective, experience and well-being are central to any assessment of need within a family. The key message for practice is that children's rights, child-centredness and the voice of the child are essential to the delivery of safe, effective care and the achievement of best outcomes. This will be a theme throughout the book, represented especially by the recurring 'child perspective' boxes.

Parents and parenting

Safeguarding children is often promoted as being 'everyone's responsibility' but it is important to note that it is primarily the role and responsibility of parents (or others, who hold parental responsibility for, or have care of, a child). Parenting has been widely recognized as being one of the most challenging roles that anyone performs, with the least preparation. As Woolmore, in a contribution to a parliamentary review of the child protection system in England, proposed: 'If I had a magic wand, I would use it to help children and young people start understanding what being a parent is about and what the needs of young children are' (House of Commons Education Committee 2012:22). Good parenting, or even good enough parenting, can be subjective, and what is expected of parents by professionals can vary according to the family circumstances (Taylor *et al.* 2009). However, it is the impact of any parental behaviours on the child that is important in any assessment of parenting capacity (HM Government 2015a). Most practitioners would recognize that good parenting involves the provision of a warm and loving relationship, ensuring that children's health and welfare needs are met and that they are kept safe and protected. It also involves providing children with the stimulation and opportunities to learn, as well as the boundaries, stability and consistency that best support children's developmental needs into adulthood.

An understanding of good parenting is helpful for health professionals, and others, in determining what support may be needed for families by providing a benchmark for assessment of strengths and deficits, including potential risk of harm to children and young people. However, in most cases it will be the parents who will be encouraged to seek support themselves and this recognition is important in determining parenting capacity and which services (over and above universal provision) may be provided.

Practice question

What is the difference between supporting *parents* and supporting *parenting*?

Positive parenting

Adopting and promoting a 'positive parenting' approach, where good behaviour is rewarded, and bad behaviour ignored, is a strategy that can do much to improve the outcomes for children and contribute to happy and fulfilling parenting. This includes helping to prevent child maltreatment. Nurses, midwives and health visitors can help to support positive parenting, as well as signpost parents to locally provided programmes that offer a structured approach to building and developing skills. An example of one such programme is given below.

Triple P programme: positive parenting and prevention of child maltreatment

The Triple P programme[2] ('positive parenting programme') is an evidence-based initiative that is demonstrating a preventative effect with families who are at high risk of maltreating their children. Key facets of this programme include the development of children's emotional regulation and supporting and helping parents to become resourceful, independent problem-solvers. This is achieved through the use of individual and group sessions, and in the provision of materials to support learning and promote positive parenting techniques. Developed by an Australian psychologist, the programme is becoming well established across the UK.

Fatherhood

The roles and responsibilities of fathers in ensuring the health, safety and well-being of their children deserve a special mention. In the UK, the Fatherhood Institute[3] takes a research-based approach to influencing policy and practice, including practice within health care. The Institute promotes the need for improvements in paternity provision and the inclusion of fathers in the delivery of services for children and young people. This has important implications for maternity services and broader child health provision, where arguably there has tended to be a woman/mother-centred approach to care provision and delivery. As Ferguson (2012) notes, this approach can mean that men miss out on the opportunity to develop their parenting abilities and their relationships with their children. However, there are signs that progress is being made. The NSPCC supported 'Dad Project', for example, aims to help health professionals to provide information, advice and support to fathers in pregnancy and the first year of a child's life (Hogg 2014). In addition, recent legislation in England, the Children and Families Act 2014, provides a statutory basis for paternity leave and enables fathers' attendance at up to two antenatal appointments.

The Fatherhood Institute website provides details of how unmarried fathers who do not automatically have legal rights and responsibilities for their child (i.e. parental responsibility) may obtain this. There is also an explanation of why this is important in the provision of parental consent for medical procedures and in gaining access to a child's health care records. It is notable that amendments to the original legislation concerning the position of fathers and parental responsibility (as per the Children Act 1989) have sought to promote greater inclusivity, and hopefully this will continue to translate into the practice of all those working with children, young people and their families, and impact favourably on family life.

[2] http://www.triplep.net/glo-en/home/.
[3] http://www.fatherhoodinstitute.org/.

Safeguarding and child protection

The terms 'safeguarding' and 'child protection' are not directly interchangeable because the notion of safeguarding both encompasses child protection, and embraces wider activity to support the well-being of children. This can be illustrated through the provision of preventative and early help strategies, such as positive parenting programmes and additional support.

The following definition of safeguarding, which links safeguarding with promoting the welfare of children, is taken from the statutory guidance for England.[4] Here safeguarding is seen to embrace:

- protecting children from maltreatment;
- preventing impairment of children's health or development;
- ensuring that children are growing up in circumstances consistent with the provision of safe and effective care; and
- taking action to enable all children to have the best life chances.

(HM Government 2015a:92)

This definition of safeguarding reflects the move to a broader outcomes-based approach to children's policy and legislation over the past decade (as reflected in the Children Act 2004). It is a strategy that has been largely adopted in all the countries of the UK. The positive stance of the policy can be reflected through actions taken by nursing and midwifery professionals. These include prevention through the provision of help and advice to parents, as well as the promotion of healthy choices and well-being for their children. It is notable that 'safeguarding' is included as a cross-cutting theme across the model of health visiting services (DH 2012). Child protection, by way of contrast, which is part of safeguarding, reflects the actions that are carried out to protect 'specific children who may be suffering or likely to suffer from significant harm' (HM Government 2015a:92).

Practice question

In line with statutory guidance, Local Safeguarding Children Boards (LSCBs) (or their equivalent) produce local policies and procedures for inter-agency working to safeguard and protect children. In addition, each health care organization will also have its own 'in house' policy and procedures. Are you aware of how to locate and use these documents in your locality?

[4]In recognition that England has the largest population of children and young people, when compared with the other countries of the UK, this book will, for the most part, reflect English statutory guidance. The Appendix provides more details and signposts comparative documents for Wales, Scotland and Northern Ireland, albeit that there are essentially many similarities across the UK as a whole.

Risks to children's well-being

The increased risks to children and young people's health, safety and well-being associated with parental mental health difficulties, substance misuse and/ or domestic violence are widely acknowledged within contemporary policy. There is also striking evidence of these risks being greater for children of parents who have never worked, or are long-term unemployed, when compared to the children of those from professional or managerial classes. These factors have important ramifications for the commissioning and provision of equitable and accessible health services that seek to address inequalities in health. Where risk is present, it is important to balance this with known protective factors, being mindful of the impact of parental difficulties on the daily lived experiences of the child. There will be many families in which risk factors are present, but where children are not maltreated (Munro *et al.* 2014). The quality of parent–child attachment can act as a protective factor, with so called 'disorganized attachment' acting as both an indicator and a consequence of child maltreatment and parenting difficulties (Shemmings and Shemmings 2011).

Practice question

What is the role of your organization in addressing health inequalities in your locality?

Child maltreatment

Child maltreatment (also widely referred to as 'child abuse' and 'neglect') is a challenging concept to define, not least because what is, or is not, considered to be harmful to children can vary both over time and between individuals, according to their knowledge, beliefs and values (Corby *et al.* 2012). However, while an understanding of cultural diversity is an important aspect of care provision, a cross-cultural consensus about what is harmful to children should prevail (Davies and Ward 2012). Statutory guidance defines child maltreatment as referring both to the infliction of harm, and failing to take action to prevent harm (HM Government 2015a). More detail is provided in the World Health Organization's (WHO) definition, favoured by Munro *et al.* (2014):

> Child abuse or maltreatment consists of all forms of physical and/or emotional ill-treatment, sexual abuse, neglect or negligent treatment or commercial or other exploitation, resulting in actual or potential harm to the child's health, survival, development or dignity in the context of a relationship of responsibility, trust or power.
>
> (Butchart *et al.* 2006:59).

In the UK, child maltreatment is frequently categorized by policy-makers and practitioners as 'physical, emotional or sexual abuse or neglect' although in reality these forms of maltreatment overlap and may co-exist. Importantly, child maltreatment most commonly occurs within family settings with parents, or other family members, or those known to the child, the usual perpetrators. This reality is reflected in the case studies described in this book. However, child maltreatment can also occur in institutions (including hospitals) and within communities. Over the past few years the UK has also seen the emergence of so-called 'celebrity abuse', with the actions of the late Jimmy Savile being particularly newsworthy. Readers will no doubt be aware of the evidence from a raft of reviews and inquiries that has found that Savile sexually abused his victims within the NHS and other institutions (Gray and Watt 2013; Lampard 2014). Stranger abuse, although also of strong interest in the media, and a source of much anxiety to parents, is relatively rare.

Practice point

It can be helpful to consider child maltreatment as part of a spectrum of 'poor to good parenting'. Nurses and midwives, who provide care to all families, are in a position where they can make judgements that benchmark the care of children with the non-maltreating majority. However, many prefer a definition that has a more clear-cut dividing line between behaviour that is indicative of abuse and behaviour which is not. Either way, this is challenging territory and practitioners may face considerable debate with other professional or lay viewpoints when considering a possibility of maltreatment occurring within a family.

Significant harm

The context of harm and the longer term effects on the victim are important factors in the assessment of child maltreatment, especially where decisions are to be made in relation to the threshold for statutory intervention in family life – i.e. the need to invoke child protection proceedings. The concept of 'significant harm', a term introduced by the Children Act 1989 (England and Wales), is noteworthy because it recognizes the need to consider a range of factors, including:

- the nature of harm;
- the impact on the health and development of the child;
- any special needs in the child (including disability or medical condition);
- the parental capacity to meet the needs of the child; and
- the context of the family and environment.

Reflecting on the 'daily lived experiences' of the child and the 'child's perspective' can aid nurses', midwives' and health visitors' professional judgement about whether or not a child is suffering significant harm. Clinical supervision is key because this provides an important opportunity to reflect on what is happening within a family with a more senior and experienced professional and to ensure a balance of risk and protective factors are considered.

The impact of child maltreatment

Recognizing and responding to concerns about possible child maltreatment is important in terms of the major impact that abuse and neglect have on health and well-being, both in, and beyond, childhood. This can include:

- death;
- neurological damage;
- disability;
- physical injuries;
- mental health problems (including depression and self-harm);
- poor self-esteem;
- attachment disorders;
- emotional and behavioural problems; and
- educational difficulties.

There is a need to acknowledge and promote awareness of the emerging findings of a body of research in the USA that links poor health and social outcomes in adulthood with child maltreatment. While there are a small number of individuals who may show a degree of resilience to harm, the 'adverse childhood event' (ACE) population studies[5] provide a substantial evidence base to link maltreatment in childhood with the increased likelihood of smoking, alcoholism, substance misuse, depression, suicide attempts, sexual health problems, physical inactivity, severe obesity and risk of premature death in adulthood. In essence, the ACE model provides the links between child maltreatment (and other adversity in childhood) to social, emotional and cognitive impairment and an increased likelihood of the adoption of health risk behaviours (e.g. substance misuse) that in turn cause disease, disability and socioeconomic problems that may lead to an early death. From a public health (and humanitarian) point of view, it is clear that it is imperative to ensure that resources are targeted towards prevention and early response to those at risk.

[5]http://www.cdc.gov/violenceprevention/acestudy/.

The prevalence of child maltreatment

It is important for nurses, midwives and health visitors to understand the prevalence of child maltreatment, as well as its impact on the health of populations. While the UNCRC is clear that children have a fundamental right to be protected from violence, it is noted to be an 'all too real' part of life for millions of children around the world (UNICEF 2014:1) as well as the cause of a significant number of child deaths. However, as Corby *et al.* (2012) suggest, a complete and accurate picture of the incidence and prevalence of child maltreatment is unlikely to be established. A useful information source for the UK is the NSPCC's annual report entitled *How Safe are Our Children?* This currently shows welcome evidence of improvements in the experiences of children and young people, while also noting that almost one in five young people aged between 11 and 17 years surveyed reports experiencing high levels of maltreatment in their childhoods (Jütte *et al.* 2014).

Physical assault, especially non-accidental head injury, is the most common cause of maltreatment deaths, but neglect can also be an important factor. While child deaths from abuse by parents or carers are rare, and rates do appear to be declining in the UK (Sidebotham *et al.* 2012; Jütte *et al.* 2014), such deaths are pivotal in informing the direction of policy and practice, especially where they have been in the public eye. The risk appears to be greatest in infancy, although research that has considered the learning from severe and fatal cases of child maltreatment has also identified that adolescents who were abused or neglected in their early childhood can be extremely vulnerable to death from suicide and risk-taking and that this leads to a second peak in the statistics (Brandon *et al.* 2014a).

Safeguarding children and public health

Successful safeguarding children work not only improves outcomes during childhood, but also the well-being of populations. The burden of ill health and poor outcomes from adverse events in childhood, including child maltreatment, is increasingly significant in countries such as the UK, where health and well-being are generally improving. While the burden of poor health and misery in children will be foremost in the minds of the caring professions, we cannot ignore a recent finding that the cost of child maltreatment in the UK has been estimated to be £15 billion per annum (All Party Parliamentary Group 2015). Safeguarding children and young people is thus recognized as a major public health issue that requires a public health solution (WHO 2006). This point is taken up by Ferguson (2009), who notes that safeguarding is part of the continuum of care provided by a range of practitioners to families and that it sits comfortably within a health improvement model (at primary, secondary and tertiary levels of prevention). Such an approach, she suggests, builds capability and capacity and makes effective use of resources. It acknowledges that professionals, and indeed lay people, are well placed and well able to identify issues of concern about the safety and well-being of a child.

Ferguson argues that a public health approach is enabling and seeks to offer a range of practical support, training and supervision to front-line staff with clear lines of accountability. Crucially it also allows a move from a 'disease model', where 'signs and symptoms' of child abuse were identified by health specialists and responsibility passed to statutory lead agencies, to one that engenders prevention and early intervention and empowers the family and a range of practitioners to work together towards positive outcomes for children. This approach is recognized throughout this book and is one that should sit comfortably with contemporary nursing and midwifery practice.

Knowledge, skills and competencies for safeguarding and child protection practice

Thus far, this chapter has introduced some key definitions: child, childhood, parenting, safeguarding, child protection and child maltreatment. Safeguarding children has been described within a public health framework which has, in turn, given nurses and midwives a mandate for prevention and early intervention; proactive work with families in addition to their responsibilities to recognize and respond to concerns that a child may be suffering from abuse or neglect. As Daniel (2015) has suggested, the raft of formal child protection processes can make this work look complicated, but, as she adds, this is fundamentally about 'noticing and helping' children who are vulnerable or 'not happy', and that there is evidence to suggest that professionals are good at doing this. Chapters 2 to 8 of this book have been structured in a logical way that allows the processes listed below to be sequenced through the case studies that form the essence of the book:

- the use of the 'Common Assessment Framework' (CAF) or 'Early Help Assessment' (EHA);
- making a referral to children's social care services;
- strategy discussions;
- initial child protection conferences;
- core groups;
- child protection review conferences;
- child death review processes;
- serious case review processes and other learning and improvement reviews.

The case studies will demonstrate that the core attributes of nursing, midwifery and health visiting, which include good communication and assessment skills, as well as knowledge of child care and development, are important tools for high-quality safeguarding and child protection work. Practitioners also need to be confident in sharing information appropriately and in ensuring that they keep clear, concise and accurate records that demonstrate their professional decision-making. More detail on these aspects of professional practice, as well as sources of support, is provided later in the chapter. However, excellence in safeguarding and child protection is fundamentally dependent on authoritative practice, and the importance and meaning of this concept (which may be unfamiliar to some readers) is discussed below.

Authoritative practice

Authoritative practice has been described as being: 'urgent, thorough, challenging, with a low threshold of concern, keeping the focus on the child, and with high expectations of parenting and of what services should expect of themselves' (Haringey Local Safeguarding Children Board 2009:67–8). As Tuck (2013) notes, these attributes are seen to be especially important in working with families who are overtly resistant to services, or demonstrating disguised compliance, or where interventions are not providing timely, improved outcomes for children. Authoritative practice can be a difficult concept to grapple with, not least by those who understand that successful child protection practice is based on the establishment of trusting and compassionate relationships with families (Munro 2011). However, the two concepts are not mutually exclusive; as Tuck proposes, trust needs to be established with care, with the professional also able to demonstrate 'respectful uncertainty' and 'curiosity' about what is happening within a family. Knowledge of the family history, rehearsal of a contact and a sense of purpose can all help to underpin authoritative practice. In turn, clinical (child protection) supervision can help by modelling authoritative practice through robust, but supportive, challenge in relation to the impact of professional practice on outcomes for children. Authoritative supervision can thus help to avoid the 'drift' which is common in complex child protection cases. As the statutory guidance notes: 'For children who need additional help, every day matters' (HM Government 2015a:7).

Recognizing and responding to child maltreatment

Despite the wealth of studies and literature that have sought to describe and measure child maltreatment, it is widely acknowledged that it remains under-recognized and under-reported. As Jütte et al. (2014) suggest, for each child subject to a formal child protection plan, it is likely that there will be another eight children who need protection. It is concerning that health professionals have been identified as sometimes being slow to recognize maltreatment and to respond appropriately, even where there are clear signs of abuse or neglect. The reasons for this (Gilbert *et al.* 2008) may include:

- poor knowledge;
- anxiety about relationships with families;
- uncertainty about the ability of statutory agencies (i.e. social care) to respond.

Through the case scenarios, this book seeks to promote a better understanding of the child protection process as well as the features of child maltreatment. Both are important if we are to meaningfully improve practice and impact on the needless morbidity and mortality that results from child maltreatment.

Although the case studies are built on the practice of nurses, midwives and health visitors, it is important to note that this practice takes place within an inter-agency context and together with professionals from a raft of statutory and voluntary organizations. The lead child protection agencies are children's social care and the police service, and it is important to understand the roles and responsibilities of professionals from these agencies at the outset.

Local authority children's social care departments (sometimes referred to as 'children's services') have a statutory duty to make enquiries if they have a reason to suspect that a child in their area is suffering, or at risk of suffering, significant harm. The child protection social worker is responsible for making enquiries and undertaking assessments. Social workers work closely with the police in undertaking enquiries, including joint interviewing of children and young people who may have suffered maltreatment. All children and young people who are 'subject to a child protection plan' will have an allocated social worker. As well as making a leading contribution to core groups and child protection conferences, the social worker may also work closely with their legal advisers in cases which go before the family courts.

Any police officer can support the need to take action to safeguard and promote the welfare of a child or young person through the use of the powers of police protection (see Chapter 3). However, all police forces also have a dedicated team of officers who have a statutory role in child protection and safeguarding as part of their public protection duties. This will include investigating the criminal aspects of child abuse cases and working closely with colleagues from other agencies in sharing information and intelligence. Particular links are made with their work on domestic abuse and violence, and the protection of victims, including multi-agency risk assessment conferencing (MARAC) and multi-agency public protection arrangements (MAPPA). In addition, police officers are involved in all unexpected deaths.

Information-sharing and inter-agency working

The notion of liaising with other professionals and agencies can raise concerns among health care practitioners about information-sharing practices. However, successful safeguarding often relies on 'piecing together' information from a variety of sources to get a clear picture of risks and strengths within a family. Most situations of significant harm to children and young people are related to a compilation of significant events and context, rather than reflecting an 'incident'.

Information-sharing guidance for front-line practitioners and their managers providing safeguarding services to children, young people and their families has been recently updated (HM Government 2015b). This new guidance notes that a failure to record, share and understand the significance of information, and to take appropriate action, is a key factor that is highlighted in serious case reviews. The guidance incorporates the 'Seven Golden Rules of Information-sharing' that seek to help practitioners to share information appropriately, securely and within the confines of legislation. Nurses and midwives will find the guidance helpful not only in meeting their safeguarding and child protection responsibilities, but also in their wider practice. The guidance reinforces the notion that the Data Protection Act 1998 is not a barrier to information-sharing, but that it provides a framework to share information appropriately. This may include sharing information without consent where a child is at risk of, or suffering from, maltreatment (although it is good practice to normally seek consent to share unless to do so would place a child at greater risk). The guidance also notes the importance of documentation, including recording a decision not to share. In line with current policies to reduce prescription from the centre, the guidance both recognizes the importance of professional judgement and the need for locally determined information-sharing protocols and arrangements. The NMC code also supports the sharing of information in line with the relevant legislation when a practitioner is concerned that someone may be at risk of harm (NMC 2015). However, for practitioners who are anxious or uncertain it will be important to seek advice from a manager or safeguarding lead. It is also the case that emergent concerns about possible child maltreatment can be discussed with lead statutory agencies without providing the name of the child or family unless or until it becomes apparent that it is necessary to do so.

Record-keeping

Record-keeping is a crucially important aspect of safeguarding children practice. As well as records being clear, factual and contemporary accounts of the assessment and delivery of care, they should also demonstrate justification of decision-making, including that relating to sharing information with other practitioners and agencies. The professional code outlines expectations relating to written and electronic record-keeping, including the storage of data (NMC 2015).

Nursing and midwifery records may be secured in cases of serious or fatal child abuse, and they can also be used in court proceedings. Poor record-keeping is a common theme in findings from serious case reviews.[6] This includes the

---

[6]And in cases of misconduct that come before the NMC.

examples of: illegible signatures; failures of practitioners to give their designation (e.g. health visitor, community midwife, etc.); lack of clarity about assessment, decision-making, care planning and evaluation of care delivery; and, crucially, a failure to *reflect the views and wishes of the child*.

Practice question

How can you ensure that your record-keeping meets the required standard?

Safeguarding children leadership in the NHS

Statutory guidance outlines the national and local strategic leadership, improvement and assurance responsibilities of NHS England and clinical commissioning groups (CCGs) in ensuring that the health system is meeting its responsibilities to safeguard and promote the welfare of children (HM Government 2015a). An executive clinical lead from each of these organizations will have safeguarding as part of their portfolios. This will mean that they will work closely with designated professionals (see below) and LSCBs in meeting the statutory requirements.

Designated professionals for safeguarding children

CCGs are required to employ, or have a contractual agreement, to secure the expertise of designated professionals (to include designated doctors and nurses for safeguarding children and looked-after children, as well as designated paediatricians for unexpected deaths in childhood). Designated professionals provide strategic leadership and clinical expertise to the CCG, NHS England, the local authority, the LSCB and other health professionals. Arrangements may be in place for one CCG to 'host' a designated professional team that is working across a local authority area.

Named professionals for safeguarding children

All providers of NHS funded services (NHS Trusts, NHS Foundation Trusts and the public, voluntary sector, independent sector and social enterprises) are required to identify a named doctor and named nurse, and a named midwife if maternity services are provided. The role of named professionals is to promote good safeguarding practice within their organization, provide advice and support to fellow professionals and to ensure that training is in place.

Practice question

Do you know the names and contact details for your named and designated professionals?

Model job descriptions for named and designated professionals, as well as details of the levels of knowledge, skills and competences required for the broader range of health professional and support worker roles can be found in the intercollegiate guidance on safeguarding children and young people (RCPCH 2014).

Summary

This introductory chapter has outlined the principles for practice that provide the foundation for an understanding of the content and context of the book. As such it has provided an opportunity to review understanding of the key definitions of child, childhood, parenting, safeguarding and child maltreatment. The chapter has also considered the professional roles and responsibilities for nurses and midwives and introduced the child protection processes and roles of lead agencies. Child maltreatment has been highlighted as a major contemporary public health issue, but seen to be amenable to a public health solution.

Safeguarding children work is challenging and emotionally demanding. Improving knowledge and the ability to practise well is important, but I know from my teaching and supervision that this may lead some to doubt their previous judgements and actions. I would like to provide reassurance that it is very likely that those who feel this way would have done the best that they could with the knowledge they then had, within the confines of their organization's prioritization of, and commitment to, safeguarding and child protection. By reading this book, you will be in a better position to practise well.

Key points

- Safeguarding children applies to individuals from pre-birth to 18 years of age.
- Children's rights and child-centredness are essential to the delivery of safe, effective care and the achievement of best outcomes.
- Parents have the overriding responsibility to ensure that their children are safe; fathers need to be included in decision-making about and care of their children.
- Child maltreatment is a major contemporary public health issue, but it is also open to a public health solution.
- Authoritative practice can help to ensure a timely and helpful response to children who may be in need of safeguarding and protection from harm.

2
Prevention and early help

Learning outcomes

This chapter will help you to:

- Develop your knowledge and understanding of the principles of prevention and early help in safeguarding children and young people.
- Extend your nursing and midwifery skills in assessment to incorporate the use of Early Help Assessments (EHAs).
- Take a role as a lead professional working with a multi-agency team around the child.
- Make a positive contribution to the safety and well-being of children through proactive practice that includes early help and family empowerment.
- Understand the key components of the Family Nurse Partnership (FNP) programme.

Introduction

This chapter concerns the practice roles of nurses, midwives and health visitors in prevention and early help in safeguarding children and young people. Three case scenarios are presented, and alongside these the rationale for nursing and midwifery actions. While the cases reference the roles of a family nurse, a health visitor and a school nurse, the mandate for prevention and early help is one for wider professions as well.

The cases are as follows:

- Case 1: Erin who is 16 years old, in care and newly pregnant. Erin is referred to the FNP programme.
- Case 2: the Gordon family, who are facing difficulties in parenting their young children and receive additional support from a health visitor including an EHA.
- Case 3: Natalie, who is 15 years old and is facing pressure from her boyfriend to be more intimate. She attends a school nurse 'drop in' session.

These cases are rooted in universal provision of health services – i.e. midwifery, health visiting and school nursing – although reference is also made to other key players such as the general practitioner (GP). Throughout the chapter links are given to policy and the evidence base for practice. There are also practice questions and points as well as suggestions for additional activities to encourage readers to further develop the knowledge and skills required for achieving excellence in safeguarding children practice.

Early help

The use of the term 'early help' is gaining prominence in describing the identification and response to emerging problems in childhood, where information-sharing and a shared approach to assessment aims to ensure that families receive the right services, at the right time, to help prevent needs becoming more acute and difficult to meet (HM Government 2015a, 2015b). It recognizes that there are a range of services for children, young people and their families, and that where there are concerns it is important for all public sector agencies to work together to address these, with children's social care only becoming additionally involved with those at the highest level of need or risk (Jütte *et al.* 2014).

The use of the term 'early help' reflects Munro's (2011) argument that 'help' carries a stronger connotation of working with families and supporting their aims and efforts to change than the more commonly used 'early intervention'. Importantly, Munro adds that this does not take away from the fact that child protection work requires authoritative (see Chapter 1), and at times coercive, action to protect children and young people from harm.

Although 'early help' can be provided for problems at any stage of childhood (from unborn to 18 years of age) there has been a recent cross-party policy directive that specifically looks at the importance of the period from conception to 2 years of age; the so-called '1001 critical days'. This directive has sought to require local authorities, CCGs and Health and Wellbeing Boards to prioritize prevention and the promotion of infant mental health, well-being and secure attachments to help to prevent child maltreatment; with early help integral to the recommendations (All Party Parliamentary Group 2015).

Case 1: Erin - support from the Family Nurse Partnership programme

Erin, who is 16 years old and a 'looked-after young person',[1] is attending a prenatal booking clinic run by Sarah, a midwife with a special interest in teenage pregnancy. Erin has had a series of placements since she was taken into care at the age of 11 following a sexually abusive relationship perpetrated by her mother's boyfriend from which her mother was unable to offer her protection.

[1]The term 'looked-after' was introduced by the Children Act 1989 and refers to children subject to care orders and children accommodated by voluntary agreement of their parents. This group is now usually known as 'children in care'.

Erin is attending the clinic with her current foster mother, who appears to be supportive. Erin has not seen her biological father for some years and has no siblings. Recently she has stopped attending college where she was studying for a National Vocational Qualification (NVQ) Level One in beauty therapy. Her foster mother stated that Erin had been doing well at college, and in addition to the NVQ was retaking her mathematics General Certificate of Secondary Education (GCSE) having only narrowly missed getting a grade C the first time around. Erin is reluctant to disclose the identity of the baby's father and says that although he is aware of the pregnancy and seems pleased by it, they are not really in a stable relationship. Sarah is concerned about Erin's vulnerability, preparedness for the baby and her ability to parent. She refers Erin to the FNP programme.

 Child's perspective

There are two children to consider in this case: there is the unborn child whose needs for optimum maternal well-being in pregnancy are self-evident, and Erin herself is also a child, and will be experiencing a range of emotions – joy, fear and bewilderment. It will be important that her views are respected and listened to, and that she is able to play an active role in determining her care and her preparations for birth and beyond. Her own experience of child sexual abuse and of loss of family are important considerations in assessment and care provision.

Teenage pregnancy

Teenage pregnancy is acknowledged to be both a cause of, and to result in, social exclusion and poverty. Rates of teenage pregnancy have been recognized as a key indicator of inequality within the Public Health Outcomes framework for England and monitored as part of the health improvement domain. The health risks to teenage parents and their offspring are well-documented. For example, teenage mothers are three times more likely to smoke in pregnancy, to suffer from postnatal depression, to be not in employment, education or training, and be less likely to breast feed (DH 2013). Fathers tend to be teenage or in their early twenties. Young fathers are themselves more likely to have suffered child maltreatment; to be suffering from anxiety, depression or conduct disorders; to drink, smoke or misuse substances; and to have poor health and nutrition (DCSF/DH 2009). Widely known risks for babies born to teenage parents include higher infant mortality and morbidity, pre-maturity, low birth weight, poor educational outcomes and greater likelihood of being unemployed in later life. Nevertheless, it is important to recognize that the poorer outcomes and the greater risk of maltreatment can also be linked to the poverty and social deprivation suffered by this group and that many babies born to teenage parents do well and achieve good outcomes.

> ## Summary of the risks and outcomes for babies born to teenage mothers
>
> - Preterm birth.
> - Low birth weight.
> - Higher rate of morbidity and mortality.
> - Poorer educational outcomes.
> - Increased risk of suffering child maltreatment.
> - Greater likelihood of being unemployed in later life.

Although the rates of teenage pregnancy are declining in the UK, the country continues to have one of the highest teenage pregnancy rates in western Europe (DH 2013). The factors that contribute to this, as well as possible solutions, remain subject to public scrutiny and polarizing viewpoints. According to the Teenage Pregnancy Knowledge Exchange (TPKE),[2] there are a number of factors that need to be in place at a local level to prevent teenage pregnancy, including:

- support for parents to discuss relationships and sexual health;
- advice and access to contraception in non-health youth settings;
- sex and relationship education in schools.

Comparisons of the UK rates of teenage pregnancy are frequently made with the Netherlands. The Netherlands has a more liberal relationship-based approach to sex education, more accessible contraception and sexual health services and teenage pregnancy rates that are one-fifth of the rates in the UK. However, despite the wealth of evidence many remain ambivalent about the mandatory provision of sex and relationship education within educational or home settings, with notable resistance from some faith-based groups.

Practice question

Reflect on your position on sex and relationship education and contraception provision to children and young people. How could this influence your practice?

Teenage pregnancy, looked-after children and young people

Looked-after children and young people are known to be at significantly increased risk of poorer health and educational outcomes, including a higher

[2]http://www.beds.ac.uk/knowledgeexchange.

risk of teenage pregnancy (NICE 2010; RCN/RCPCH 2015). In a summary of the evidence base to support this finding, the Social Care Institute for Excellence (SCIE) concluded that this was not only because the health, education social and economic difficulties and disadvantage were more prominent within this group, but also because the young people suffer from having limited access to positive adult support and yet are expected to be more independent (SCIE 2005). The SCIE review also suggests that because of educational disadvantage, including poor attainment and attendance, looked-after children and young people were unlikely to benefit from either school-based sexual health and relationship programmes or the provision of school-based contraception and sexual health services. Drawing on consultation with young people, the review highlighted the options for greater accessibility to confidential sources of information and advice on sexual health matters, such as through social media and the internet, as well as the need for provision of specialist sexual health services for this age group.

Practice point

Despite the negativity that surrounds teenage parenthood, it is important for nurses and midwives to acknowledge that parenthood is a familiar 'rite of passage' and may serve to provide meaning to individuals with poor self-esteem and self-worth whose childhood has failed to allow them to achieve their potential into adulthood.

Sarah's post as a midwife with a special interest in teenage pregnancy is an example of work undertaken within the NHS to try to address young people's reported anxiety about the possible reactions of health professionals to teenage pregnancy and their additional concerns about receiving maternity care alongside older service users (DCSF/DH 2009). Sensitivity to the needs of teenage parents and provision of bespoke services to meet these needs can help to ensure better outcomes for their children and address the intergenerational cycle of deprivation that can ensue.

Activity

Access You're Welcome: Quality Criteria for Young People Friendly Health Services (DH 2011) from the Department of Health (DH) website (www. dh.gov.uk). This initiative aims to help in the planning and delivery of high-quality and 'young-person friendly' health services.

•   How does your service measure up?
•   What can you do to make a small and sustainable improvement?

Case 1 continued

During the booking appointment, Sarah discusses the options for Erin's care in pregnancy with her. Although Erin's foster mother is keen to contribute and be involved in the planning for the new baby, Sarah ensures that she spends some time with Erin alone. This provides an opportunity for a more sensitive discussion about her pregnancy and her relationship with the father of the baby, and to ensure that if possible he is able to join Erin at future appointments. Sarah also recognizes the need to consider and explore any possibility of coercion, sexual exploitation and/or sexual abuse, especially given Erin's vulnerability, disengagement from education and her initial reluctance to disclose details about the father (HM Government 2009). Once Erin is comfortable with Sarah she will also engineer an opportunity to see her alone to address any issues of domestic (intimate partner) violence or abuse. She may also approach the issue of a return to education and recommend that the family find out about the 'Care to Learn' benefits which have been introduced to encourage teenage parents to complete their education. Sarah concludes the appointment by asking Erin where she would like to receive her care and what the best times for her future appointments might be. They discuss the use of texting to keep in touch to help with any queries and to send new appointments. Finally Sarah gives Erin a positive message in letting her know that she is eligible for the help and support of a practitioner from the FNP programme.

The Family Nurse Partnership programme

The FNP programme[3] is an evidence-based intensive scheme for young (typically under the age of 19) and vulnerable first-time mothers. It comprises highly structured scripted home visits by specially trained nurses (generally experienced health visitors and midwives) and is delivered from the prenatal period until the child is 2 years of age. The programme is based on the Nurse Family Partnership programme first trialled in the USA in the late 1970s. Participants in the programme have been rigorously followed up in a series of robust randomized controlled trials that have shown significant improvements in the life chances of the mothers and their children, with concomitant savings to the public purse.

FNP focuses on improving outcomes, so that teenage mothers are able to:

- have a healthy pregnancy;
- improve their child's health and development;
- plan their own futures and achieve their aspirations.

[3]http://fnp.nhs.uk/.

The structure of home visits focuses on health-promoting behaviours and self-efficacy skills that will improve outcomes for the mother, child and wider family. FNP seeks to encourage and support access to contraception and sexual health services and education, and promote opportunities to gain employment and build supportive relationships with family members and friends. The practitioners who deliver the programme, known as 'family nurses' receive regular one to one and group supervision.

The key differences between FNP and the universal Healthy Child Programme (DH/DCSF 2009a) are that there is continuity of practitioner from the antenatal period until the child's second birthday and that there are more contacts. Family nurses receive additional training that supports delivery of strengths-based approaches aimed at increasing clients' skills, confidence and hope for the future.

Evidence of the success of the programme in the USA can be summarized as:

- measurable improvements in maternal and child health;
- reduction in children's injuries, illnesses and hospital admissions;
- reduction in child maltreatment;
- improvements in school readiness and educational achievements;
- reduction in substance misuse;
- fewer subsequent pregnancies and greater intervals between births;
- less criminality by the young mothers;
- increase in fathers' involvement;
- increase in maternal employment; and
- reductions in spending on welfare.

In short, the programme demonstrates both improved outcomes for children, young people and families, and cost benefits to the public purse (Olds et al. 1994, 1997; Eckenrode et al. 2010). However, because of the difference in health and social care systems in the UK, and especially in the provision of universal midwifery and domiciliary health visiting services, it is acknowledged that the effects of FNP may not be directly comparable to the clear indicators of success in the USA (Ball et al. 2012). Nevertheless, emergent evidence suggests that early adopter sites have been able to demonstrate acceptability of the programme, together with a range of encouraging outcomes including a positive impact on smoking reduction and increased rates of breast feeding, as well as being a positive experience for those nurses and midwives who have become family nurses (Barnes et al. 2009; Ball et al. 2012). Importantly, the programme is recognized to be a good example of a targeted service provision within the universally provided *Healthy Child Programme* (DH/DCSF 2009a) and as an intervention that has the potential to reduce health inequalities in vulnerable populations.

Practice question

How can targeted care within universal services be delivered to ensure that those who receive additional services gain most benefit without a sense of being stigmatized?

Erin: summary of prevention and early help

For Erin, if the outcomes of FNP mirror those in the USA (albeit with the proviso given above) the baby will be more likely to be born at term within the normal range for birth weight and to be breastfed. The baby may also have an increased likelihood of being healthier with a reduced possibility of suffering illness, an accident or maltreatment, and may achieve greater success at school. Erin will be more likely to return to college to obtain her qualifications, gain employment and have a longer gap before a subsequent pregnancy. The father of the baby will be more likely to be involved in their care.

Markers of good practice: the role of the midwife

Sarah, who has specialized in teenage pregnancy, understands that Erin and her baby face a risk of poor health outcomes. As a highly skilled and knowledgeable practitioner, Sarah is able to begin to establish a positive and trusting relationship with Erin and is able to arrange a programme of care that will meet her needs and wishes.

Sarah is able to negotiate some time to see Erin alone and will make a particular assessment of any evidence of maltreatment, including sexual exploitation. She will also assess for domestic (intimate partner) violence and abuse.

Case 2: the Gordon family – assessment of additional needs using an Early Help Assessment

Marlon and Kay are the parents of two boys, Maddox aged 22 months and Mason aged 6 months. Kay, who has mild learning difficulties, is finding it hard to cope with the needs and demands of a baby and a toddler. Marlon often threatens to leave because he 'can't stand the babies crying'. He is currently unemployed although had previously been working in a small local business as a storeman. Both parents smoke cigarettes but deny the use of other substances. The family are living in a privately rented two bedroomed flat which is difficult to heat and often feels damp. They are concerned about the threatened cuts to housing benefit.

Kay rarely sees her mother, who lives on the other side of the city. She has few friends and finds going out difficult as Marlon is not prepared to look after the children for very long. Kay has been feeling low since the birth of Mason who was born at 32 weeks' gestation due to maternal infection. Jenny, the health visitor, is concerned about Kay's ability to meet the needs of her boys. Maddox appears to be behind in his developmental milestones and has recently missed an appointment with the community paediatrician. He often appears somewhat grubby and is usually sucking on a dummy (pacifier) while trying to hold onto Kay's legs. Mason has not yet completed his primary course of immunizations and has been somewhat poorly following an episode of bronchiolitis. There are concerns that he is failing to gain weight as expected.

Jenny, who has been offering an enhanced service with extra home visits, is concerned that without additional services the children may end up suffering from neglect of their health and developmental needs. She is also aware that both parents are trying to do their best but are limited by their circumstances and abilities. Jenny seeks the consent of Marlon and Kay to identify their needs by undertaking an assessment using the locally determined 'Early Help Assessment' (EHA) process.

 Child's perspective

The impact of parental difficulties is having an adverse effect on the health and well-being of Maddox and Mason. These children are living with parental discord and it is very likely that this will be affecting their emotional well-being and sense of security. Maddox has missed a crucial appointment to have his development assessed. The use of a dummy and a lack of positive engagement, stimulation and communication from parents will almost certainly be impacting on his development of speech and language skills. Mason is physically unwell, and is compromised by missing out on immunizations. His preterm birth makes him additionally vulnerable and his poor weight gain reflects his physical illness, but could also be a result of under-feeding. If the parents are smoking cigarettes in the house then these children are at risk from the effects of passive smoking (Royal College of Physicians 2010).

Early Help Assessment

EHA builds on the creation of a common assessment framework (CAF) developed as part of the Every Child Matters policy stream (DfES 2004). The EHA is a voluntary process. Recent policy promotes the importance of early help and encourages local areas to develop a range of early help provision. This includes the ownership of local assessment processes (HM Government 2015a). Reflecting the centrality of the child and the importance of an ecological approach to assessment, the three domains 'child development', 'parents and carers' and 'family and environment' are examined within the model or framework. Thus, EHAs will typically make an assessment of the following:

Child development	Parents and carers	Family and environment
Health and emotional well-being	Basic care	Family history and functioning
Behaviour development	Ensuring safety and protection	Wider family
Relationships	Emotional warmth and stability	Housing
Social skills	Guidance, boundaries and stimulation	Employment and financial elements
		Social and community elements

Any front-line practitioner can undertake an EHA. The reason for doing so should be made clear and the assessment balanced. This means identifying both strengths and needs, and being open and honest with the family about emergent worries and concerns. While it is acceptable to have a 'professional opinion', providing evidence to support a viewpoint is mutually helpful. Parents and, where age and developmentally appropriate, children and young people will give informed consent for the completion of an EHA, and for any information-sharing within and across agencies that is necessary for any additional services to be provided. Where consent is not given, it will be for the practitioner to make a judgement as to whether or not it is necessary to take further action to safeguard and protect the child.

The EHA is normally electronically enabled (i.e. available as an online tool) to ensure that the assessment planning and review elements are securely shared and updated. E-enablement can help in the strategic planning of services by making it easier for local authorities to analyse the demographics of families who have had an EHA and are in receipt of additional services. The development of multi-agency safeguarding hubs (MASHs) where services are co-located can also support the EHA process by ensuring appropriate and timely sharing of information and provision of the right help at the right time.

In representing the dynamic and changing nature of needs within families it is important to note that movement takes place across a continuum of need; however, the aim is always to take early action to support movement towards minimal intervention in family life and return to universal provision of services. In some cases, it may be appropriate to run through a 'pre-EHA' checklist that acts as an aide memoir to make a rapid assessment of a child's safety and well-being. Where additional needs are identified through the EHA these may be able to be met by one practitioner, with the assessment acting as a focus for what needs to happen to ensure the health and well-being of the child. It is essential that the child, parents and wider family are also brought into the plan, thereby building capacity for families to help themselves and be solution focused. Where the needs and service provision are more complex, an involved practitioner will take on a role as a 'lead professional' to act as a single point of contact for the family. Nurses and midwives from a range of specialties may take on this role, although most commonly this would be the health visitor. Equally, it may be more applicable for another professional – for example, from the youth offending team or a special educational needs coordinator (SENCO) to do so. The lead professional ensures that the child or young person and their family receive appropriate and timely interventions. This includes coordinating a plan outlining outcome-focused actions for the team and family, and ensuring that these are delivered and reviewed in a planned way that reduces the possibility of duplication or overlap. Where others need to be involved, a 'team around the child' (TAC)[4] meeting, involving the child, family and professionals, will help to ensure good join-up of services and delivery of the plan.

If an EHA has been completed it is a useful adjunct to a referral to children's social care services (or indeed any other service) providing that appropriate information-sharing protocols are followed. However, in my experience, there appears to be some confusion in practice as to children's social care services' expectations of EHA completion as part of the referral process. *Working Together* is clear that while a completed EHA may be helpful in supporting a referral it is 'not a prerequisite' (HM Government 2015a:16).

Activity

Visit your local authority website and find out more information about EHAs and services in your locality.

A qualitative study to evaluate the impact of the CAF (the precursor to EHA) on the outcomes for children, young people and their families suggests that there is some evidence to show improvements in children's physical and emotional health, financial support and housing (Easton *et al.* 2010). Participants in the study included children, young people and their families as well as practitioners from the children's workforce. Midwives, health visitors and school nurses were among those drawn from health agencies. In addition to the indications of better outcomes for children, the study also noted improved integrated working and trust between agencies. However, the authors concluded that more work was needed to ensure that the outcomes achieved were sustainable.

Case 2 continued

The evidence suggests that the children of parents with a learning disability may be more likely to have developmental delay and that any delay may be compounded by a potential for lack of stimulation within their environment

---

[4]Some areas refer to this as a 'team around the family' or TAF.

(Gaw 2000). Although Kay's learning disability is thought to be mild, it is important that those providing care to the family are sensitive and appreciate that the impact of detailed assessment may add to a common fear within this group that their children may be removed from their care. Before starting the assessment Jenny seeks consent, ensuring that Kay and Marlon understand the nature of the EHA and how the information that is shared may be stored and used. She also provides reassurance that the process will help to identify where parenting is going well in addition to discovering what else may be needed to ensure that the boys are able to achieve their health and developmental potential.

Jenny thinks that at the current time the needs of the family can be met through some targeted support and monitoring provided by the health visiting team and children's centre. The EHA action plan includes the following.

For the parents:

- to attend Maddox's appointment with the paediatrician to assess for developmental delay;
- to agree to a referral for Maddox to attend the speech and language therapy service;
- to take Mason to the GP to complete his schedule of immunizations;
- to attend the Thursday drop in parent and toddler group (a volunteer from the group will come and meet the family at home to befriend Kay);
- for Kay to see the GP to discuss postnatal depression;
- for Marlon and Kay to address their contraception and sexual health needs;
- for Marlon and Kay to seek help from the local smoke-stop service; if they continue to smoke they will do so on the balcony of the flat and not in front of the children.

For the health visiting team:

- the health visitor to make an application to an early years scheme that supports nursery placements for vulnerable 2-year-olds;
- the nursery nurse to undertake a programme of weekly visits to model suitable play activities for both boys;
- the health visitor to arrange an invitation for the parents to attend a parenting group at the children's centre;
- the health visitor to write to the local housing officer to support a move into more suitable accommodation for the family.

The Gordon family: summary of prevention and early intervention

The decision to undertake the EHA was based on the evidence that the children had unmet health and developmental needs and the understanding that early help may help to avoid issues reaching crisis point. Plans to meet the additional needs were put in place. The situation will be reviewed in due course; if there is evidence that unmet needs remain, additional services may be required. However, if concerns about the neglect of the two children continue, or escalate, then it will be necessary to refer the case to children's social care services for a statutory assessment.

Markers of good practice: the role of the health visitor

Despite offering an enhanced service, Jenny recognizes that the Gordon family has a number of unmet needs that are impacting on the health and development of the children. In line with best practice guidance in working with parents who have a learning disability, Jenny is careful to explain the nature of the assessment, mindful that research has found that such clients can feel negatively judged and discriminated against (DH/DCSF 2007). With consent from the parents an EHA is completed. This recognizes some strengths and positives within the family, but also enables the completion of an action plan to ensure that unmet needs are addressed.

While feeling sympathy for the parents, Jenny will ensure that her focus remains on the 'daily lived experience' of the children and will escalate her concerns to children's social care if necessary.

Case 3: Natalie – prevention and support from the school nursing service

Natalie is a quiet and studious 15-year-old who has recently become involved with Hunter, a mature student at the nearby university, whom she met at the local leisure centre. Her father is a civil engineer and her mother works part-time at a local nursery school. She has a younger brother who is due to join her at her secondary school the following academic year. Natalie is concerned that her family would disapprove of her friendship with Hunter and has begun to meet him secretly while telling her parents that she is working in the library after school. Hunter has had previous relationships and is putting pressure on Natalie to be more intimate. She is aware that other students in her class are involved in sexual relationships with their boyfriends and is anxious that she is not seen to be a bit of a 'geek' with no life outside her studies; indeed, she has already received some unpleasant messages from classmates on Facebook. Natalie believes that if she does not agree to sleep with Hunter he will end their relationship. She is becoming increasingly anxious and withdrawn. At a recent parents' evening, that Natalie also attended, her form tutor expressed concern that she seemed unhappy and that her grades had slipped over the previous term. In an effort to continue the relationship, Natalie arranges to stay overnight at the halls of residence, telling her parents that she is having a 'sleep-over' at her best friend's house. Knowing that the school nurse, Cynthia, is able to provide contraception and sexual health advice, Natalie decides to attend a lunchtime drop in session.

Underage sexual activity

In the UK, the 'age of consent' is 16 years. Sexual activity before this age could be considered to be unlawful, although it is widely recognized that legal action is unlikely for consensual sex of those aged 13 years or over with a partner within their age group. The same rules apply whether the activity is heterosexual or homosexual. Prosecution will be more likely the larger the age gap, or where there is an imbalance of power, or an individual has a position of trust or authority (e.g. a health professional or teacher).

Practice question

What advice and support would you give to a 15-year-old seeking contraception and sexual health advice in the following circumstances? Do any of the following circumstances require a referral to lead agencies?

- Their partner was 18 years of age.
- Their partner was 28 years of age.
- They were reluctant to disclose details of their partner.
- They appeared to have a learning difficulty.
- They were accompanied by an older adult who didn't disclose their relationship with the young person.
- They looked younger than their stated 15 years.
- They said they were 'coming for a friend'.
- They disclosed use of alcohol and/or other substances.

Case 3 continued

At 15 years of age, Natalie believes that she is in a minority within her peer group because she is still a virgin. However, recent evidence from a wide-ranging survey of sexual attitudes and lifestyles in the UK (Natsal-3)[5] found that 29 per cent of women aged 16–24 years reported that they had sexual intercourse before the age of 16 years. Hunter is 25 years old.

[5] http://www.natsal.ac.uk/.

Practice question

Should Cynthia, the school nurse, be considering sharing information with children's social care and/or the police?

School nurses working in 'drop in' sessions with children and young people will be working within the remit of the professional code (NMC 2015). In establishing a rapport, it will be important for Cynthia to ensure that Natalie understands the issues in relation to consent and confidentiality. Specific guidance to support school nursing in the provision of sexual health and relationship advice outlines the role of the school nurse as one of promoting confidence and emotional resilience in young people and helping them to understand the benefits of loving, healthy relationships, and in delaying sex (DH 2014). The guidance also helps practitioners to consider whether contact needs to be made with safeguarding or child protection services.

Cynthia considers that Natalie is presenting as a vulnerable young person who is at risk of harm. While letting Natalie know that she has been sensible to 'drop in' to discuss contraception, she shares her concerns that Hunter is considerably older than she is, and that she may be being coerced into a sexual relationship before she is ready. Cynthia also explains that the secret nature of their relationship is particularly worrying and adds that because Natalie (and others) may be at risk from Hunter's predatory behaviour she would like to share information about him with other agencies (police and social care). Cynthia also encourages Natalie to be more open with her parents, while assuring her of the confidentiality of the health aspects of the consultation, in particular that her personal information will not be shared with her parents or the school. Finally, she advises Natalie that the majority of 15-year-olds are unlikely to be engaging in sexual activity whatever her classmates say. Natalie is visibly relieved.

 Young person's perspective

Natalie is experiencing a number of stressors – an older boyfriend, who is putting pressure on her to have sex, some bullying from classmates on social media and pressure from parents and the school to do well in her academic studies. At the same time she will be experiencing the rapid, and sometimes confusing, changes of adolescence in her physical, sexual, social and emotional development. Having access to sexual health advice in school is important to Natalie – and the 'drop in' nature of the service has helped to prevent her from being coerced into a sexual relationship before she is ready.

Natalie: summary of prevention and early intervention

Underage sexual activity is unlawful and can be a serious cause of concern. Even where it is consensual, there may be serious consequences to the welfare of the young person, including unplanned pregnancy and sexually transmitted infections. Where there is a clear imbalance of age or power this needs to be considered as 'sexual exploitation' with a clear risk of significant harm to a young person or other young people (see Chapter 6). Information may need to be shared with statutory agencies (i.e. children's social care and/or the police) and this should be explained to the young person and where possible their consent gained to do so. The actions of the school nurse will protect Natalie's well-being and potentially add to intelligence about an individual who poses a predatory threat to young girls.

Markers of good practice: the role of the school nurse

Cynthia runs a confidential 'drop in' session to support the health needs of young people in a place and at a time to suit them. The aim is to promote health and well-being, especially in relation to physical, emotional and sexual health.

While acknowledging the step that Natalie has made in consulting with her as a sign of maturity, Cynthia has also recognized Natalie's vulnerability within a relationship which is marked by secrecy and an imbalance of power. Cynthia seeks supervision and support from the named nurse safeguarding children (see Chapter 1). She then contacts the local children's social care department, which in turn, contacts the police. Cynthia completes clear, contemporaneous records of her decision-making and actions (NMC 2015).

Summary

This chapter has applied the principles of prevention and early help in safeguarding and promoting the welfare of children to nursing and midwifery practice. It has described how targeting services within a universal service (i.e. the FNP, enhanced health visiting, and proactive school nursing) can help to prevent the development of more serious concerns about children and young people. The case scenarios have shown the importance of the assessment skills of the practitioners. Through considering Cynthia's actions, the chapter has also demonstrated that the actions of nurses and midwives can have a significant impact on the wider health and safety of children and young people. Some prevention and early help activity will take place at a 'single agency' level. However, much of what can be achieved is also reliant on working in an integrated way with other professionals and agencies. This will be explored in more detail in the other chapters of this book.

Key points

- Midwives, health visitors and school nurses have a range of opportunities to contribute to the prevention and early identification of child abuse and neglect.

- The FNP may confer a range of improved outcomes for the most vulnerable families including a reduction in child maltreatment.

- The EHA process provides a framework to assess strengths and needs within a family and to ensure timely support.

- Those providing contraception and sexual health services need to practise within the framework of legislation and guidance. This will include supporting children and young people's safety, as well as their health.

3

Physical abuse

Learning outcomes

This chapter will help you to:

- Understand the features of physical abuse as a form of child maltreatment.
- Identify indicators that may be associated with physical abuse, including fabricated and induced illness.
- Outline the key components of nursing assessment, paediatric examination and investigations in cases of possible physical abuse.
- Understand the process for referral of cases of suspected child maltreatment to the lead statutory agencies (children's social care and/or the police) and the purpose of the strategy discussion.
- Appreciate the role and functions of the named nurse safeguarding children and the local authority social worker.

Introduction

This chapter considers physical abuse as a form of child maltreatment. Physical abuse can present in many different ways and may be difficult to distinguish from accidental injuries (sometimes referred to as 'non-intentional'). This chapter does not aim to be inclusive of all possible presentations. However, what it does aim to do is develop nurses', midwives' and health visitors' understanding of how this form of child maltreatment may present; the factors that may help to inform its identification and referral; and what the nursing actions should be. The aim is to ensure that children and young people are safeguarded and protected from further harm in a timely and appropriate way.

Drawing on the statutory guidance we define what is meant by 'physical abuse' and outline some of the key indicators of concern. Three case scenarios are presented, together with the nursing actions. The cases are as follows:

- Case 1: Kayla, aged 10 weeks, who is visiting the practice nurse for her first immunization. A bruise is noted.

- Case 2: Ethan, aged 14 months, who has attended the emergency department with two small burns on his hand; he is noticed to be somewhat withdrawn.
- Case 3: Naimah, a 6-year-old, who has been admitted to a children's hospital for investigations of chronic diarrhoea.

The cases are fictitious, but based on real events. As in the previous chapter, reference is made to safeguarding children policy, as well as the underpinning evidence for practice. We begin by providing a brief overview of the features of physical abuse. The chapter concludes by summarizing key practice points to help to reinforce knowledge and best practice.

Physical abuse

The definitions provided in *Working Together* for the purposes of statutory child protection proceedings and planning are a useful starting point in helping those working with children, young people and their families to understand child maltreatment and its presenting features (HM Government 2015a). Here, four 'categories' of maltreatment are referred to: physical abuse, emotional abuse, sexual abuse and neglect.

Physical abuse is described as involving: 'hitting, shaking, throwing, poisoning, burning or scalding, drowning, suffocating or otherwise causing physical harm to a child. Physical harm may also be caused when a parent or carer fabricates the symptoms of, or deliberately induces, illness in a child' (HM Government 2015a:92). The finding from a respected national survey (Radford *et al.* 2011) that 7 per cent of 11–17-year-olds report serious physical abuse during their childhood is widely quoted within the field.

Children and young people who become subject to a multi-agency child protection plan in one of the four categories outlined above are considered to have unresolved safeguarding children issues and to remain at risk of significant harm. While overall numbers of children subject to a child protection plan have been rising over the past few years, the percentage of children who are subject to a plan under the category of 'physical abuse' has fallen disproportionately to account for around 10 per cent of the total numbers (DfE 2014a). The figures are not in themselves indicative of the incidence or prevalence of this type of abuse, but do help to demonstrate that, perhaps in contrast to public opinion, physical abuse is not a leading cause of statutory intervention.

It is notable that 'hitting' is included in the statutory definition of physical abuse. The issue of the legality of physical punishment blurs the boundaries between what some would consider acceptable treatment of children and others abusive (Polnay *et al.* 2007). While rates of corporal punishment in the UK have declined in recent years (Jütte *et al.* 2014), it remains a global issue of concern (UNICEF 2014). At the time of writing, the UK has yet to join the 44 countries around the world that have instigated a ban on hitting children, despite the fact that nursing, midwifery and health visiting professional organizations have indicated their support to do so.[1]

Female genital mutilation (FGM) is a form of violence that that has a significant impact on the physical and emotional health of victims (HM Government 2014; DH 2015). FGM relates to 'all procedures involving partial or total removal of the external genitalia or other injury to the female genital organs for non-medical reasons' (RCM *et al.* 2013). The WHO describes FGM as a practice that is deeply rooted in inequality between men and women. FGM is illegal in the UK and should be viewed and responded to as a form of physical child abuse. Its proponents believe that it promotes fidelity and chastity and may promote it on the basis of cultural expression. Dean (2014) notes that nurses (e.g. school nurses and practice nurses), midwives and health visitors are in a good position to identify and refer children at risk of FGM to lead statutory agencies. Recent guidance signals an intention to make reporting mandatory (HM Government, 2014; DH 2015).

Practice points

FGM is prevalent in many different cultures and communities.

FGM can be carried out at any time in childhood; however, the peak age is when the girl is between 5 and 8 years old.

Children may be at risk of being taken abroad by their families for a 'special procedure'.

FGM is associated with urinary tract problems, sexual health problems, infertility and complications in pregnancy. It also has psychological effects.

Routine enquiry by health professionals is advocated and value-neutral terms should be used (e.g. 'Have you been closed/circumcised/cut down there?').

(Adapted from Dean 2014)

Severe and fatal physical abuse

At the severe end of the spectrum, physical abuse can lead to permanent disability or death. Infants are particularly at risk. The NSPCC provides a helpful explanation of how child maltreatment death statistics are gathered. It has updated the widely reported previous estimates of one child fatality per week (in England and Wales) by including the reviews of the serious child care incidents that are reported to the Office for Standards in Education (Ofsted). As a result of this work, the NSPCC now suggests that up to three children die

[1] http://www.childrenareunbeatable.org.uk/.

as a result of maltreatment each week, but that this may be an underestimate (NSPCC 2014). While such tragedies may occur in circumstances where there are no apparent prior indicators of maltreatment, a history of escalating concerns about physical injuries and other indicators of abuse or neglect (such as a context of substance misuse or domestic violence) are a feature of many serious case reviews, albeit with the benefit of hindsight. Identification of possible non-accidental (or 'intentional' or 'inflicted') injuries or patterns of injuries is thus an important professional role and responsibility for nurses, midwives, health visitors and others in contact with children and their families.

Recognizing physical abuse

It is helpful to begin this section by reflecting on what has recently been described as the 'art and science' of child protection work; here recognizing maltreatment is seen to be 'dependent on the trigger of an initial index of suspicion, supported by a mix of corrobative detail, experience, triangulation, monitoring, review and above all the highest level of multi-agency communication and co-operation' (Cass 2014:101). Nurses, midwives and health visitors are not expected to 'diagnose' child maltreatment; this normally requires a child protection medical assessment, combined with robust history-taking, the gathering of contextual detail and deliberations with statutory lead agencies. However, in common with a number of front-line practitioners working with children, young people and their families, nursing and midwifery staff are expected to be able to recognize presentations that raise concerns about the possibility of child maltreatment and to take action accordingly (RCPCH 2014; NMC 2015). The NICE guidance (NCCWCH 2009) provides an essential resource to support practitioners who are concerned about a child. The guidance is set out in a way that outlines when maltreatment should be *considered* as a possible explanation for a presentation for health care, and when it should be *suspected* and where a referral to children's social care may follow.

Practice point

Children who are developmentally able should be encouraged and supported to provide their own history for a presenting injury. They should also be given an opportunity during a consultation to be seen without the accompanying parent or carer. The approach should always aim to be 'child centred'.

Identifying possible abuse is dependent on history, context and clinical indicators. The NICE guidance (NCCWCH 2009) offers a helpful interpretation of how a judgement may be made regarding an unsuitable explanation for an injury or presentation – i.e. one that is 'implausible, inadequate or inconsistent'

(p. 23). This can relate to the presentation, normal activities, existing medical condition, age or developmental stage of the history presented by parents. Inconsistent explanations between parents or carers, or those that change over time, are also seen to be a marker of concern. However, as Sidebotham (2015) has argued, it is not unusual to obtain a changing history in practice due to a range of factors that include fear and anxiety on the part of parents, as well as the skills and experience of the clinician. NICE guidance also cautions against accepting an injury or presentation as being related to a cultural practice or religious belief as this does not justify harming a child.

The following case scenarios describe three different presentations of physical child abuse. Links are made to the evidence base for practice and to statutory guidance. In each case, the actions of the nurse are described in terms of best practice.

Case 1: Kayla – an infant with bruising

Kayla, who is 10 weeks old, is attending an appointment with the practice nurse, Laurel, to have her first immunization. She is the first baby of Lucie and Mark, who have been together for a year or so in a somewhat volatile relationship. Kayla is a small baby, having been born at term, but with a birth weight of 2479 grams. She is fed on infant formula milk and has just begun to smile. As she prepares to give the vaccine, Laurel notices a small fresh bruise on Kayla's upper thigh. Lucie is unable to provide an explanation for the bruise, and in undertaking a further assessment of the baby, Laurel finds a further bruise on Kayla's back.

Practice point

Evidence from a robust controlled study suggests that breast feeding may have a protective effect against maternally perpetrated child maltreatment (Stratheam et al. 2009). This is thought to be due to the release of oxytocin which, in turn, is associated with mood elevation and reduction in stress in breast-feeding women.

Bruising

Bruising is the most common presentation of physical abuse (NCCWCH 2009). However, accidental bruising in children is also very common and it is thus important that nurses and midwives have an appreciation of presentations of bruising that may be indicative of physical abuse. The NCCWCH clinical guidelines are particularly helpful and conclude that where there is bruising in babies and children who are not independently mobile, and no clear history of an accidental cause is given, practitioners should suspect non-accidental injury (i.e. maltreatment). In comparison, independently mobile children and young people will sustain accidental bruising in everyday activities – for example, in

Table 3.1 Bruising

Non-accidental bruising	Accidental bruising
• Unexplained/no history given	• Explanation/history provided
• Bruising in babies	• More common in summer months
• Bruising in a child who is not independently mobile	• Bruising in an independently mobile child
• Bruises on any non-bony part of the face or body including eyes, ears, cheeks, upper arm, outer thigh and buttocks	• Bruises on the knees, shins, elbows, forehead, nose, centre of chin, back of head
• Bruises on the neck that look like attempted strangulation	
• Bruising in the shape of a hand, ligature, stick, teeth marks, grip, implement	
• Multiple bruises or clustering of bruises	
• Bruises with petechaiae	
• Severe bruising on the scalp accompanied by swelling to the eyes (as a result of hair pulling)	

Source: adapted from NCCWH (2009) and WCPSRG/NSPCC (2012)

play and sporting activities. Table 3.1 compares some key features of accidental and non-accidental bruising.

Although guidelines as to how to 'age' a bruise have been published in the past, the evidence for this is not conclusive and current advice is that it should not be attempted.

Case 1 continued

The presence of any injury in an infant is concerning and may suggest more serious injury. Kayla is only 10 weeks old. The next step for Laurel, the practice nurse, is to raise her concerns with Lucie and to explain that Kayla will need to be seen by a paediatrician and that a referral to the local authority children's social care service will be made. A body map may be used to indicate the position of the bruises.

In some areas, the paediatrician will see the child prior to the referral to children's social care and in others this will be arranged in conjunction with children's social care (according to local policy and procedures). Referrals to children's social care are normally made by telephone in the first instance and followed up in writing within 48 hours, usually on an inter-agency referral form designed for this purpose. Lucie, Kayla's mother, should be fully informed about the referral to children's social care, unless doing so would place Kayla at increased risk of harm. The practice nurse will need to carefully document her findings and actions, including any explanation for the injury that is offered by Lucie. In a very small minority of cases, there will be a medical explanation for the bruising.

Raising the possibility that an infant or child may have been deliberately harmed is challenging. However, the duty of care is first and foremost to the child, who is totally dependent on others to recognize the possibility of maltreatment. Every practice situation calls for communication on an individualized basis. Laurel should both seek to find an explanation for the bruises and be clear that bruising in a small baby is unusual and can indicate that *someone* may have harmed Kayla. She will explain that because of this Kayla will need to be seen by a paediatrician and be referred to children's social care.

It is also good practice to inform the GP of the situation at the earliest opportunity. However, the practice nurse is independently professionally accountable for her actions (NMC 2015). The practice has a responsibility to ensure that Kayla is taken for further assessment and to provide relevant details to those making child protection enquiries. Finally, the practice nurse should ensure that the health visiting service is made aware of the referral, according to local arrangements for primary care liaison.

Practice point

There should also be concern about the welfare of Kayla's mother, Lucie, as domestic violence and abuse is indicated. Children living with domestic abuse are at a notably increased risk of physical abuse and other forms of child maltreatment (Stanley 2011).

Referral to children's social care

Further details of the process of referral to children's social care can be found in both the statutory guidance (HM Government 2015a), guidance for practitioners (HM Government 2015c) and LSCB inter-agency procedures. As we noted in Chapter 1, each health care organization should also have its own safeguarding children policy and procedures, including details of how to contact safeguarding leads for advice and support in the identification and referral of concerns about possible child maltreatment. When a referral has been made, children's social care will liaise with the police, who will have a responsibility to progress any criminal investigation arising from safeguarding children concerns.

The sharing of information is an important part of the process and information from the GP and the health visitor will provide context for the child protection enquiries (HM Government 2015b). Support and advice for health professionals who are concerned that a child has been abused or who need help with progressing a referral to children's social care can be obtained from named professionals and their team. The police should be notified of any situations that may further endanger the child, for example parental refusal to comply with the requirements for their child to be seen. The Children Act 1989 has a provision known as 'police protection' (Section 46) that allows a police officer to either move a child to a place of safety or prevent a child being taken from a place of safety. Police protection can last for up to 72 hours.

Case 1 continued

Kayla will have a comprehensive paediatric assessment and medical examination. As she has presented with bruising this will include investigations to exclude the possibility of bleeding disorders or meningococcal septicaemia, which may look like bruising. The paediatrician will also take a full family and social history, and document the findings carefully. This will include taking details of who has had care of Kayla (which will also be part of the police and social care enquiries). The bruises will be recorded on a body map and may be photographed by a medical or forensic photographer.

Kayla is a small baby, and the assessment will include a measurement of her current weight and plotting of previous known weights, including her birth weight, on a 'centile chart'. Previous weights (and other health details) should be available in the 'parent-held child health record' (widely known as the 'red book'). Lucie will be asked to share this record with the professionals undertaking the assessment.

Children who suffer physical abuse may also show signs of neglect. A key indicator of neglect is a failure of growth along expected centiles (see Chapter 7). Kayla is reported to have *just* started to smile. This is later than expected (normally 6 weeks of age) and may suggest developmental delay (Sharma and Cockerill 2014).

Practice point

Those who provide care to infants, children and young people should be familiar with key developmental milestones. Child maltreatment is one of the possible causes of developmental delay in children (Polnay *et al.* 2007).

In cases of suspected physical abuse of infants under the age of 12 months, a skeletal survey will normally be undertaken to see if fractures are also present. According to NCCWCH (2009) guidelines, non-accidental fractures are more common in infants and toddlers and may also be 'occult' – i.e. not clinically evident on physical examination. Some fractures, especially metaphyseal or rib fractures, can occur without bruising (WCPSRG/NSPCC 2012). The skeletal survey provides a standard series of images that enable the whole skeleton to be visualized (Royal College of Radiologists & RCPCH 2008). As with blood tests, it is important that Lucie and Mark (assuming Mark has parental responsibility – see Chapter 1) are informed of the rationale for undertaking this investigation, which is essentially to exclude the presence of disease or other injuries.

A further key concern is the possibility that Kayla may have sustained a non-accidental head injury. Non-accidental head injury is the commonest cause of death in physical child abuse and most commonly presents in infants younger than 6 months of age. Given the presentation of bruising in a young baby, neuroimaging in the form of a computerized tomography (CT) scan may be ordered to check for any evidence of non-accidental head injury.

 Child's perspective

At 10 weeks of age Kayla is entirely dependent on her parents to meet her needs. She may be feeling pain and hunger, accompanied by fearfulness. There are already signs of disorganized attachment (Shemmings and Shemmings 2011).

Possible investigations for suspected non-accidental injury

- Full blood count and clotting studies.
- Skeletal survey.
- CT scan.
- Forensic photography .

Kayla: summary of concerns

Kayla was noted by the practice nurse to have bruising to her upper thigh and back. Bruising in an infant is highly indicative of physical maltreatment and may indicate a risk for more serious injury. The practice nurse, seeing Kayla for a routine immunization, took action to address her concerns with the mother and to make a referral for further paediatric assessment and enquiries by children's social care.

Markers of good practice: the role of the practice nurse

As a practitioner who has responsibility for seeing infants and children for care, including immunizations, Laurel is familiar with child care and development and has a good understanding of indicators of possible child maltreatment.

> Laurel is aware that bruising in an infant who is not independently mobile is indicative of physical child abuse, especially in the absence of an explanation.
>
> Laurel correctly refers the case to children's social care, informs the GP of her concerns, and explains to the child's mother that further paediatric assessment and examination will be required. She will follow up her telephone referral to social care in writing, and liaise with the health visitor.
>
> Laurel completes clear, contemporaneous records of the events and her actions (NMC 2015).

Case 2: Ethan – a toddler with burns

Ethan, aged 14 months, is taken to the emergency department by his father, who has care of him during alternate weekends and for one night each week. Ethan has two blistered areas on his hands, said to be caused by offering him food that had been reheated in the microwave (the suitability of a microwave for heating baby and toddler food and drinks remains open to debate, however, it is common practice and appropriate advice should be given about 'hot spots' and testing food.) One of the areas looks as though it is infected. Ethan has been to the emergency department on four previous occasions and, as had been noted on the most recent visit, he appears to be somewhat withdrawn and quiet. Michael, an emergency nurse practitioner, is allocated to care for Ethan and his father.

Thermal injuries

According to the WCPSRG (2014) most burns and scalds are accidental, with approximately 10–14 per cent of burns seen in children admitted to specialist burns units thought to be a result of an intentional (non-accidental) injury. However, neglect to provide for the safety of a child is an important contributory factor in many additional cases, and this would include failure to protect a child from sunburn. Burns are painful, potentially lethal, and can cause lifelong scarring and psychological damage (NCCWCH 2009).

Safety advice: prevention of burns and scalds in children

- Set the thermostat on hot water systems to a maximum of 50°C.
- Ensure safety when ironing, cooking and making hot drinks.
- Remove cigarette lighters and matches from children's reach.
- Provide additional protection from the sun for babies and young children (i.e. more than for an older child or adult).

As with bruising, there are some features or patterns of thermal injury that may raise suspicion as to the possibility of child physical abuse. These include (NCCWCH 2009:31–2):

- the presence of upper limit or symmetrical scalds on the extremities;
- glove or stocking pattern of injury;
- an isolated scald on the buttocks, perineum or lower extremities;
- a scald that is uniform in depth, where flexures are spared, or in the case of immersion;
- co-existing other injuries, including fractures;
- previous burn injury;
- burns on a not independently mobile child;
- burns or scalds that are in the shape of an implement.

In any presentation of physical injury it is important to also consider late presentation, whether the history is compatible with the explanation given, the general appearance of the child, previous medical and social history (including any concerns about siblings) and current family and social circumstances. A lack of parental concern, or the presentation of the child by an unrelated adult are important indicators of the possibility of non-accidental injury. The WCPSRG review group has drawn up a useful colour-coded triage tool that can be uploaded to help to support decision-making in distinguishing between accidental and intentional scalds (WCPSRG 2014).

Practice point

Each year up to 50 per cent of infants and 25 per cent of older children present to an emergency department or urgent care centre. Children account for some 25 per cent of all emergency department attendances. Clinical staff working in these areas need to be competent in caring for children and young people. This will include having skills in child development, communication with children and young people, as well as safeguarding and child protection (RCPCH 2012).

Case 2 continued

Ethan and his father will be seen promptly for triage and treatment, including pain relief as appropriate. Registration details will include noting who the health visitor is (or which health visiting team is responsible for Ethan's care) and contact may be made directly with the liaison health visitor according to local protocols to ensure rapid exchange of health information. Michael, the emergency nurse practitioner, will also note the relationship of the accompanying adult(s) and seek to address any immediate concerns and queries that they have (RCPCH 2012). Michael will access the details of previous attendances at the emergency department (and ask about attendance at other centres, for example minor injury/walk in facilities). He will make a full health assessment (including body weight), establish a developmental and social history and conduct a full and comprehensive examination for the presence of other injuries. Michael will also ensure that a check has been undertaken to see if Ethan is currently subject to a child protection plan.

In respect of this presentation, Michael will ask for details of the timing and mechanism of the injuries and cross-check with any explanation that has been given to colleagues in triage. Findings will be recorded, and a body map completed. Michael will seek the opinion of a senior medical practitioner, either a paediatrician or a senior doctor in emergency medicine. The most concerning aspect of this presentation is the fact that both hands are blistered. At 14 months of age Ethan will be keen to try out his sense of touch and be developing his fine motor movements and reach. He will also be attempting to feed himself. However, he would be unlikely to place *both* hands in hot food.

It is likely that Ethan will be admitted to the children's ward. Good practice dictates that children should not be discharged while concerns remain about their safety or well-being (Laming 2009). A referral will be made to children's social care, as per Kayla's case (Case 1). Because of the concerns that this is a non-accidental injury, a social worker will convene and lead a formal strategy discussion.

Strategy discussions

A strategy discussion, led by children's social care and involving senior practitioners from the police, health staff and other relevant professionals (e.g. nursery or school staff) should be convened whenever there is 'reasonable cause to suspect that a child is suffering, or is likely to suffer significant harm' (HM Government 2015a:36). Rapid action may be needed and the discussion will normally be held within one working day of a concern coming to light, and more than one strategy discussion may be required. The role and importance of health professional input has been reflected in the latest guidance. In an emergency the discussion may be held over the telephone, although this can limit the contribution of the participants and the rich discussion that results from a face-to-face meeting. Where a child is in hospital it is expected that the medical consultant in charge of the child's care attends, along with a senior member of the ward's nursing team. Where a child has needed specialist care (e.g. from an orthopaedic team), then their involvement may also be key. In practice, this might mean a paediatrician reporting on their behalf. If a parent is experiencing problems such as domestic violence, substance misuse or mental health problems, then a professional from one of the supporting services may also be involved in the strategy discussion.

Practice point

Where a child is an inpatient, ward staff are well placed to comment on interactions between children and their parents and carers. Nursing and midwifery staff should be supported at strategy discussions by a safe-guarding children specialist such as a named nurse.

The purpose of the strategy discussion is to:

- share information about the nature and context of the concerns;
- agree the timing and conduct of any criminal investigation;
- make a decision on the need to undertake child protection enquiries;
- ensure the immediate safety of the child (and any other children in the family); and
- discuss what information will be shared with the family (unless to do so would increase the risk to the child or other children or jeopardize any criminal investigations).

Those contributing to the strategy discussion will need to ensure that information-sharing and decision-making reflect the best interests of the child, and that the outcome of the meeting includes plans to ascertain their wishes and feelings. Strategy discussions should be chaired by the representative from children's social care and minuted.

Child's perspective

Ethan will be frightened and in pain. He is reliant on the skills and knowledge of the emergency department professionals to provide a response to his inflicted injuries. Ethan is in unfamiliar surroundings, and will be seen by a number of unfamiliar adults. Ensuring a child-friendly environment, with the provision of age-appropriate toys and paediatrically trained staff (including a play specialist) will help to make his experience of attending hospital less daunting.

Ethan: summary of concerns

Ethan has sustained burns to both hands, representing a symmetrical injury to extremities that is not consistent with developmental expectations. Furthermore, the fact that one of the burns looks infected may suggest a delay in presentation. The fact that Ethan has previous attendances at the emergency department, as well as his demeanour, adds to concerns. This presentation needs to be treated as a child protection concern.

Markers of good practice: the role of the emergency nurse practitioner

Children and young people represent approximately one-quarter of all attendances in the emergency department, and it is thus important that those practising in this setting are competent in the delivery of care. If a nurse working in an area that treats children does not hold a children's nursing qualification they should work under the supervision and guidance of a registered nurse (child), until they are deemed competent in the delivery of care to children.

As an emergency nurse practitioner, Michael is responsible for the care and assessment of a number of children and young people each day. His experience has informed his expertise in recognizing a sick child – i.e. his awareness of developmental milestones and the range of behaviours and interactions between children, young people and their parents.

Michael undertakes a comprehensive assessment of Ethan. This includes a full, detailed history and examination. He also checks Ethan's child protection status, and re-reviews details of the previous attendances.

Michael considers that there had been some delay in the presentation of Ethan, and is also concerned about the child's demeanour and senses wariness between Ethan and his father.

Michael is also of the opinion that the history of the injury is incompatible with the findings. He discusses his assessment and concerns about possible maltreatment with his senior and a paediatric opinion is sought.

Michael will complete a notification form for the attention of the liaison health visitor (with details of the attendance). He will also complete the written referral to children's social care and attend the strategy discussion.

Michael completes a clear, contemporaneous record of the events and his actions.

Case 3: Naimah – a 6-year-old in hospital

The final scenario in this chapter concerns the special challenges of caring for a child and family where there are concerns that indicate that the child is presenting within the 'spectrum' (RCPCH 2009) of illness behaviour that may indicate fabricated or induced illness (FII). Naimah, who is 6 years old, has been admitted to a ward in a specialist children's hospital. This is her fourth admission and, as before, she is accompanied by her mother who wishes to be resident. Naimah is a bright girl, but her education is suffering due to frequent absences from the classroom. Naimah's parents are divorced and she is their only child. Her father works abroad in the oil industry and her mother, Ariana, is a full-time mother and housewife, who previously completed two years of an advanced diploma in nursing (adult branch), failing to progress to the final year because of her own ill health.

Naimah has been admitted because of her mother's continuing concerns about her abdominal pain and loose stools, reporting that sometimes she has up to six episodes of diarrhoea in a day. A number of investigations have already been performed including tests to rule out infection and coeliac disease. Naimah has also been treated with an antispasmodic medication and several courses of metronidazole. To date no diagnosis has been confirmed. Naimah's mother is pleased to recognize Sally, the ward sister, whom she considers empathetic and caring.

Naimah was born at 32 weeks' gestation, her mother – who describes 'poor personal health' – having previously suffered a number of miscarriages. As a baby Naimah was reported to have lactose intolerance and required special infant formula feeds. As a toddler she was presented to her GP with reports of skin allergies. This proved difficult to treat and Ariana sought further advice from a number of complementary medicine practitioners, including several consultations with a herbalist.

Sally reviews the records and admits Naimah to the ward. Since she knew that Naimah was returning for more investigations, Sally has expressed disquiet about the possibility of FII. She feels that Naimah is essentially a well child, whose frequent presentations for health care and investigations are concerning. The admitting paediatrician agrees to a full review of the past medical history and will consult with the Trust's named professionals for safeguarding children.

Practice point

In his review of the circumstances of the death of Victoria Climbié, Laming (2003) coined the term 'respectful uncertainty' to describe an approach to ensure that professionals' assessments accurately determine the lived experience of the child. This seems to be especially important in FII where perpetrators normally enjoy good relationships with health professionals.

Fabricated or induced illness

FII is a recognized form of child physical abuse (HM Government 2015a) and, as such, the focus of the care and treatment should always be on the safety and well-being of the child or young person. It is important that all health professionals are both knowledgeable about, and alert to, the risk of this somewhat rare form of maltreatment, while recognizing that it is best understood as occurring as a possibility within a spectrum of presentations of children for health care. Bass and Glaser (2014) helpfully describe FII as being located on a continuum of parental help-seeking behaviour, from extreme neglect at one end, to actively inducing illness at the other. In some cases, suspected FII can cause tensions within and between health care teams who may be divided as to the possibility that parents or carers, who appear devoted and concerned, could deliberately harm their child. The need for support, supervision and debrief is important, as is the need to refer cases of possible FII to the lead statutory agencies in line with statutory guidance.

FII is a term that is used to describe the fabrication of physical or mental illness or disability in a well child by misconstruing or exaggerating the severity of a known condition or by deliberately inducing illness symptoms. According to the NICE guidance (NCCWCH 2009), the challenges to diagnosing (or confirming) FII include the reality that the symptoms that are described or induced are found in many common childhood illnesses, and that in some cases FII occurs *alongside* genuine conditions.

Bass and Glaser (2014:1414) refer to 'deception by the use of hands' to include falsification of records, interfering with specimens or lines (e.g. adding salt, sugar or blood) or by induction of illness through suffocation or poisoning. Perpetrators, they note, may also promote a 'sick role' or withhold medication or treatment to worsen symptoms in a known illness.

Parents, particularly mothers, are the most common perpetrators of FII, although others in a familial caring role may be implicated. In some cases, there is collusion between parents. Intergenerational transmission of this form of physical abuse has also been recognized (Bass and Glaser 2014). Perpetrators are typically described as being knowledgeable and plausible in their portrayal of the child's condition, with up to one-third having a background in health care. Many perpetrators will have their own history of childhood maltreatment.

Practice point

Midwives need to be alert to the possibility of women inducing miscarriage or preterm birth. They may also falsify their past obstetric histories or present with pseudocyesis (false pregnancy).

FII is a relatively rare condition (RCPCH 2009), but it is important in that it can cause children to undergo unnecessary, and often unpleasant, investigations and treatment, including surgery. FII can also lead to significant physical, behavioural and psychological problems for children, including confusion and anxiety about their health and adoption of a 'sick role'. Children and young people of all ages can be affected, although there is a preponderance of younger children and infants. For older children, there may be frequent absences from school and a lack of opportunity to take part in normal childhood activities, such as sport. Some victims may be made to use a wheelchair (Bass and Glaser 2014).

In severe cases FII can lead to permanent disability or death. It can take an average of nearly 2 years to identify children who may be suffering from this type of maltreatment, with an average age at diagnosis of 4 years, and boys and girls equally affected (NCCWCH 2009). There are recognized links with an increased risk of other forms of physical abuse and/or neglect both prior to, and subsequent to, diagnosis (RCPCH 2009). Bass and Glaser (2014) suggest that doctors should seek to find out what is really wrong with the child as soon as they feel 'perplexed'. This may of course be difficult to do when the vast majority of parents genuinely seek to have their child's best interests met.

Bass and Glaser (2014) summarize the literature concerning factors that may lead to fabrication or induction of illness in a child or young person. This includes parents:

- displaying extreme anxiety, leading to exaggeration to confirm a diagnosis;
- seeking to confirm a false belief about an illness in their child;
- demonstrating attention-seeking behaviour;
- deflecting the blame for a child's difficulties (e.g. a behavioural problem);
- seeking to maintain closeness with their child;
- using their child's condition for material gain.

Case 3 continued

The team looking after Naimah makes a decision to review all previous records and to seek information from others who have had care of Naimah. The consultant paediatrician takes on a role as the responsible lead paediatrician to ensure that an accurate diagnosis is made. They will also ensure that the need for further tests and procedures is minimized to avoid the possibility of 'iatrogenic harm'[2] while the review is conducted (RCPCH 2009). Best practice dictates that, in such cases, the child and family are cared for by senior team members, with careful management of confidentiality and support for the team. Sally, the ward sister, is thus allocated to manage Naimah's nursing care. In line with supplementary statutory guidance on the inter-agency management of suspected FII (HM Government 2008a), children's social care are contacted, and it is possible that they already hold information about the family that may contribute to the review.

The lead paediatrician seeks Ariana's consent to request all previous health records, as a means to 'get to the root of the problem' (RCPCH 2009). Records in such cases are normally kept secure, to avoid tampering. Charting of symptoms, such as pain or diarrhoea, will need to be explicit and verified – i.e. date, time, reported by, witnessed by, child's view of events. The Trust's

---

[2]The term 'iatrogenesis' refers to unintentional harm or complications that arise from health care investigations or treatment.

named nurse, Mei (see Chapter 1) is asked to draw up a comprehensive health chronology that will detail all of Naimah's contacts with health services.

In aiming to be focused on the safety and well-being of the child, it is important to ensure that their views and/or perspectives are provided. A fully integrated chronology drawing on data from primary and community care, as well as secondary (and any tertiary) care, will help to get a fuller picture of the possibility of FII. It is important to remember that most children will have genuine illness at some point during their childhood. An example of a template that can be used in this instance (and also for the purpose of serious case review, see Chapter 8) is given below.

Date	Time	Source of information/ professional	Description of event	Views of the child	Reviewer's comments
12/08/14– 15/08/14		Hospital records Paediatrician	Re-referred by GP with reports from mother of continued loose stools and weight loss Jejeunal biopsy Abdominal X-ray Bloods Urine screen – all 'no abnormalities detected' (NAD)	Seemed settled in hospital Noted to be a little pale and quiet, reluctant to mix with other children	Mother resident and helping with care; stool chart incomplete?
6/07/14		Letter to GP from allergy specialist	Private appointment Mother reports child has wheeze and rash To return for skin tests	No history of wheeze given on previous attendance	
14/04/14	17:35	GP records	Mild sore throat: antibiotics prescribed as child reported to have been pyrexial and very unwell over the weekend		Verification of history?

Producing a chronology is time consuming, especially in cases where there has been a multiplicity of contacts with health care agencies. However, chronologies are incredibly valuable in helping to determine causes for concern about the possibility of FII. In my experience, health data can be held in various locations and in separate case notes, even within the same health care organization. Furthermore, it is well known that perpetrators of this form of physical child abuse may 'doctor-shop' across a range of public and private health care providers. The RCPCH (2009) guidance promotes the helpfulness of the use of one set of records for children and young people, including combining the nursing and medical records and this practice was previously recommended by Laming (2003). The increasing use of electronic solutions for care recording and management will be beneficial, especially where care is accessed on a number of sites.

In considering the 'spectrum' of illness behaviour, the following are possible findings and outcomes for Naimah:

- Reassurance that there is no apparent clinical diagnosis; primary and community health professionals will arrange support to manage mother's anxiety.

- Advice in terms of what may be considered to be 'normal' in relation to daily bowel habits and encouragement for Naimah to be independent in toileting.

- Liaison with the GP, who will make a referral for the mother to be seen by adult mental health services.

- Discharge without a firm diagnosis and the possibility that a return of symptoms will lead to further interventions.

- Discovery that the symptoms reported by the mother cannot be verified by nursing records; mother also found to be falsifying charts.*

- When challenged on the basis of the chronology and review, the mother admits that she has been administering large doses of laxatives to Naimah.*

Naimah: summary of concerns

Naimah has been readmitted to hospital with a history of reported ongoing gastrointestinal problems with no clear diagnosis. There are possibilities that Ariana has fabricated aspects of the reported illness, and nursing staff have been asked to draw together a detailed chronology and ensure that accurate records are kept.

---

*These findings will mean a child protection referral is made to children's social care.

Markers of good practice: the role of the named nurse safeguarding children

As a named nurse working in a specialist children's hospital it is likely that Mei will have been involved in previous cases of suspected FII.

Mei offers support and guidance to the team caring for Naimah, and helps to coordinate the retrieval of records from various health care agencies. She offers particular guidance and support to Sally.

Using a template, Mei pulls together a detailed chronology of all Naimah's contacts with health services. The completed chronology is extensive and runs to 36 pages.

Mei ensures that professionals involved in the case are aware of the supplementary guidance on management of FII (HM Government 2008a) and local LSCB procedures.

At the conclusion of the review, and after appropriate referrals have been made, Mei arranges for a debrief session for involved professionals. This needs careful handling and should reflect the benefit of hindsight to avoid undue professional distress.

Child's perspective

As a victim of FII, Naimah is likely to be anxious and confused. She will require therapeutic intervention from a specialist CAMHS team to help her to develop a 'narrative' (Bass and Glaser 2014) about her experiences and to accept her 'wellness'. Naimah has missed out on school, friendships and a host of normal childhood activities. She may be feeling trapped within a disordered maternal–child relationship. She also misses her father, who is estranged from the family and working abroad.

Summary

This chapter has considered physical abuse, which can involve causing physical harm by deliberately injuring a child or by fabricating or inducing illness. The statutory processes of child protection referral and strategy discussions were also introduced. Although most physical abuse may be classified as being 'minor' for research and statistical purposes (it will not feel 'minor' to the victim), in severe cases, this form of abuse can lead to permanent disability or death. Serious case reviews may highlight a pattern of progressive injuries over time, which, with the benefit of hindsight may suggest missed opportunities to recognize physical maltreatment. Nurses, midwives and health visitors have a role and responsibility to identify children and young people who may be suffering from, or at risk of, physical abuse.

The three scenarios presented included non-accidental bruising in a young baby, deliberate burns in a toddler and a case involving a young girl that may prove to be FII. They are not intended to be inclusive of all types of physical abuse but demonstrate the importance of nurses', midwives' and health visitors' roles and responsibilities in recognizing and responding to child maltreatment. Apart from Mei, an experienced children's nurse and health visitor, who now specializes in safeguarding children, the nurses in this chapter see a wide range of children, young people and their families. This, together with a child- and family-centred approach to assessment, and openness to the possibility of child maltreatment, helps them to identify children and young people who may be at risk of, or suffering from, harm and to ensure their safety.

Key points

- Nurses and midwives who see children in the course of their practice should be familiar with child care and development and have a good understanding of indicators of possible child maltreatment.

- Health visitors and school nurses should be informed of all attendances at emergency departments/minor injuries units.

- A liaison health visitor/children's nurse can support information-sharing processes (two-way) between hospitals and community teams.

- Children attending for urgent care should have their child protection status checked.

- Children's social care and the police are the lead agencies for referral of child protection concerns; telephone referrals to children's social care should be followed up in writing within 48 hours.

- Clear, contemporaneous records of events and actions should be kept.

- In cases of suspected FII a robust chronology detailing all contacts with health professionals should be drawn up.

- Support and advice on any aspect of safeguarding children can be obtained from named and designated professionals.

4

Emotional abuse

Learning outcomes

This chapter will help you to:

- Understand the features of emotional abuse as a form of child maltreatment.
- Identify indicators that may be associated with emotional abuse, including significant risk factors, such as domestic violence and abuse.
- Reflect on the potential safeguarding and child protection contribution of 'adult-centred' practitioners.
- Make a practical professional contribution to an initial child protection conference.
- Understand the role of the educational welfare officer.

Introduction

This chapter considers emotional abuse and the actions that nurses, midwives and health visitors can take to ensure that children and young people who may be suffering from emotional abuse are identified, and that appropriate help and support is provided. Emotional abuse takes many forms; what is important here is that the maltreatment is likely to be contextual, rather than reflect an 'incident' (i.e. as compared to physical abuse). This means that nurses, midwives and health visitors who are providing ongoing care to a child, young person and their family are better placed to identify this form of maltreatment when compared with colleagues in more acute settings. Three practice-based scenarios will be discussed as a means of illustrating how nursing intervention can be critical in ensuring the safety and well-being of children who may be subject to emotional abuse.

- Case 1: Poppy, aged 6 years, has been referred to CAMHS because of increasingly challenging behaviour. Her mother describes her as a child who is 'difficult to love'.
- Case 2: Tyra, aged 13 years, is the oldest child in a family of four children. Tyra's school attendance has been steadily declining and there are

concerns that her parents' substance misuse difficulties have spiralled out of control.

- Case 3: Nilay, aged 9 years, suffers from severe cerebral palsy. He has recently been losing weight and has just had a procedure for a percutaneous endoscopic gastrostomy (PEG) feeding tube to provide enteral nutrition support.

As in the previous chapter, these examples are not intended to offer a fully comprehensive description of all the possible presentations of this form of child maltreatment. However, the cases do aim to provide insight into how emotional abuse may present in practice and the steps that nurses (including those whose role is primarily with the parent) should take to respond. Building on the knowledge gained about the referral process to children's social care, and the subsequent strategy discussion to share information and context for concerns, this chapter introduces the initial child protection conference (ICPC). The aim here is to help you to understand your role in contributing your nursing expertise to the conference and how decisions made at this multi-agency meeting plan for the future safety and protection of the child (or children in the family). Where the conference decision is to make a child subject to a statutory 'child protection plan' there will normally be specific actions within the plan for health professionals, especially those from universal services (i.e. midwives, health visitors, school nurses). These may include monitoring compliance with other health service provision, for example a child's attendance at a paediatric clinic or a parent's concordance with a substance misuse treatment programme. We begin by defining emotional abuse.

Emotional abuse

The *Working Together* (HM Government 2015a) definition of emotional abuse offers a good understanding of the possible presentation of this form of maltreatment. Importantly, this definition also recognizes that emotional abuse, by its very nature, is a feature of all types of child maltreatment. As we noted in Chapter 3, the statutory definitions provided in the guidance are used to categorize the type of abuse for the purpose of child protection proceedings. After concerns about child neglect (see Chapter 7), emotional abuse is now the second most common reason for children and young people to be made the subject of a child protection plan – currently running at 35 per cent of the total (DfE 2014a).

The *Working Together* definition of emotional abuse is as follows:

The persistent emotional maltreatment of a child such as to cause severe and persistent adverse effects on the child's emotional development. It may involve conveying to a child that they are worthless or unloved, inadequate, or valued only insofar as they meet the needs of another person. It may include not giving the child opportunities to express their views, deliberately silencing them or 'making fun' of what they say or how they communicate. It may feature age or developmentally inappropriate expectations being imposed on children. These may include interactions that are beyond a child's developmental capability, as well as overprotection and limitation of exploration and learning, or preventing the child participating in normal social interaction. It may involve seeing or hearing the ill-treatment of another. It may involve serious bullying (including cyber bullying), causing children frequently to feel frightened or in danger, or the exploitation or corruption of children. Some level of emotional abuse is involved in all types of maltreatment of a child, though it may occur alone.

(HM Government 2015a:92–3)

According to Davies and Ward (2012:32) emotional abuse may be 'the most damaging of all forms of maltreatment' because it directly impacts on a child's fundamental needs to be loved and nurtured. They note that this form of abuse usually overlaps with neglect, suggesting that parents' neglect of a child's basic needs is indicative of the fact that they do not understand or care about them. However, they add that emotional abuse can occur in the context of a child who is physically well cared for.

Nurses and midwives are likely to see children and young people at risk of, or suffering from, emotional maltreatment in the course of their work. This is because the risk factors for emotional abuse, which include parental mental health difficulties, substance misuse, domestic violence and abuse, family relationship problems, social isolation and disability or chronic illness in the parent or child, feature in families who are likely to be accessing health care in a variety of settings.

Practice question

How can your assessment of child and family health needs help to identify the impact of parental difficulties on the child?

Parenting and emotional abuse

Identifying emotional abuse can be difficult, and it is widely believed that those cases that are identified as such by agencies represent only the 'tip of the iceberg'. One of the challenges is that this form of abuse is almost exclusively perpetrated by parents (or those in a parenting role) and that there is a very broad range of approaches to parenting and child care behaviour that may be seen in the course of practice. While there is clearly a debate to be held as to what constitutes 'good enough parenting' (being a perfect parent is likely to be beyond the reach of mere mortals!), it is interesting to note that the literature seems to more readily outline characteristics of *poor* parenting, rather than *good* parenting. In addition, there appears to be little in the way of concrete advice for practitioners on where the line may be drawn between the two.

In one article that seeks to provide a critique of the social, economic and political context of parenting, the authors list three times as many characteristics of poor parenting, as compared to those of good parenting (Taylor *et al.* 2000). These characteristics, which might usefully inform midwifery and nursing assessment, are listed in Table 4.1.

Taylor *et al.* (2000) argue that achieving 'good enough parenting' is strongly influenced by the availability of resources and support. The authors

Table 4.1 Parenting characteristics

Characteristics of good parenting	Characteristics of poor parenting
✔ Teaching by example	• Exposure to deviant models
✔ Providing a secure environment	• Inability to provide continuity of care
✔ The mother's presence	• Poor supervision
✔ Attachment and bonding	• Lack of bonding and attachment
✔ Maturity	• Youth of the mother
✔ Unconditional affection	• Conditional affection
✔ Flexible control	• Cruel control
✔ Child-centredness	• Rejection
✔ Positive affectivity	• Negative affectivity
	• Unpredictability
	• Provocation
	• Impairment of health or development
	• Harmful or cruel discipline
	• Distance
	• Hostility
	• Intrusion
	• Poor mothering
	• Ignorance
	• Fecklessness
	• Lack of empathy for child
	• Unrealistic expectations
	• Laxity and inconsistency
	• Aggression
	• Low warmth
	• High criticism
	• Neglect
	• Abandonment

Source: adapted from Taylor *et al.* (2000:114)

express concern that while the socioeconomic determinants of the ability to parent well are evident, they are not always accounted for and that the links between poverty and adverse outcomes in childhood need to be more widely appreciated and acted on. Nurses, midwives and health visitors can be proactive in addressing inequalities in health through targeting services at those with the greatest need (i.e. ensuring needs-led, not demand-led, services). Taylor *et al.* also comment that the focus in the literature on parenting rests almost exclusively on 'mothering', and this is clearly evident in their list of characteristics above. Parenting is a shared responsibility and the father's role (as we noted in Chapter 1) needs to be both recognized and promoted.

Cultural perspectives

A further dimension in ensuring informed assessment and decision-making in safeguarding and child protection is an appreciation of the cultural aspects of family life. Polnay *et al.* (2007) usefully explore ethnicity and cultural perspectives in child maltreatment and suggest that ethnic minority families are more likely to suffer from socioeconomic deprivation as well as being marginalized within society (they describe this as a 'double jeopardy'). The authors also suggest that there are a wide range of child care practices within multicultural Britain and argue for greater thought to be given to the assessment and care of ethnic minority families to avoid different standards of care being delivered to children and young people across the spectrum.

Race and ethnicity

The issue of race and ethnicity was brought into focus in the case of Victoria Climbié. Victoria, who was born in the Ivory Coast, came to the UK via France, in the care of her great-aunt. She subsequently suffered enduring and horrendous maltreatment, perpetrated by the great-aunt and the great-aunt's partner. Victoria died, aged 8 years, on 25 February 2000. Notably, Victoria was black African, and some of the front-line workers in the case were also of black heritage. The inquiry into the case noted that:

> Assumption based on race can be just as corrosive as blatant racism. Fear of being accused of racism can stop people acting when otherwise they would. Assumptions that people of the same colour, but from different backgrounds, behave in similar ways can distort judgements.
> (Laming 2003:12)

The impact and learning from Victoria Climbié's untimely death continue to inform policy and practice.

On a practical basis, nurses, midwives and health visitors may also need to consider access to professional interpreters to ensure that care is planned and delivered in an appropriate and timely manner. It is unacceptable practice to use family members, especially children and young people, to act as interpreters in health and social care settings.

Prevention of emotional abuse

Nurses, midwives and health visitors may well have opportunities in the course of their practice to intervene to prevent emotional abuse. As Corby *et al.* (2012) note, this means active listening, empathy, sensitive challenge and supporting parents' motivation to change, with the child's experiences and well-being central to the practice encounter. It is important to be able to recognize behaviours that may be indicative of a risk of emotional abuse. Barlow and Schrader-Macmillan (2009) describe a range of possible presentations, including:

- the emotional unavailability of parents;
- the parents attributing negative intentions, beliefs or attitudes towards the child;
- developmentally inappropriate interactions;
- the parents' lack of recognition of their roles and responsibilities;
- a failure to promote the child's social adaptation.

The authors also note that positive parenting programmes such as Triple P (see Chapter 1) and targeted home visiting programmes, such as the FNP programme (see Chapter 2) may help to prevent emotional abuse because of the emphasis that these programmes place on addressing emotionally abusive parenting (anger and misattributions). They also note the benefit of joined-up working between child and adult services. This means that it is vital that practitioners understand and enact the principles of information-sharing outlined in Chapter 1 and create systems of care delivery that are truly child and family centred.

The effects of emotional abuse are widely reported to include attachment and behavioural difficulties in childhood and poor cognitive and social functioning, mental health difficulties, self-harm and suicide in adulthood. Emotional abuse may thus precipitate difficulties in childhood that may be seen to be essentially 'behavioural' (e.g. aggression, challenging behaviour, withdrawal, low achievement), although these outcomes may also reflect other forms of child maltreatment (NCCWCH 2009). In identifying emotional abuse, it is always important to consider the daily lived experience of the child or young person and to focus on the meaning of parental difficulties and deficits on their well-being.

The following scenarios describe three different presentations of childhood emotional abuse. Links are made to the evidence base for practice and to statutory guidance. In each case, the actions of the nurse are described in terms of best practice.

Case 1: Poppy – a 6-year-old child who is 'difficult to love'

Poppy is the first child of Siobhan, who has recently given birth to twin boys with a new partner. Poppy's father, Derek, who left Siobhan when Poppy was 3 years old, was known to be the perpetrator of serious domestic violence and the pregnancy was unplanned. From the outset, Siobhan found Poppy to be a difficult child; she was a colicky baby, who was difficult to settle and did not sleep through the night until she was 11 months of age. Her mother continues to describe her as a 'fussy eater'. At the time of Poppy's birth, Siobhan and Derek were living in somewhat sub-standard accommodation and were in receipt of benefits. Siobhan was just 19 years of age, and had left her childhood home and the town in which she grew up 2 years previously, following a serious disagreement with her mother. Although she has made some friends in the apartment block where she now lives, it has taken a while to build up her supportive network, and this has been aggravated by a shortage of money and difficulties in accessing child care. With a new relationship and the subsequent birth of the twins, the situation for Siobhan and the family has improved somewhat, despite the fact that the birth of twins is a significant source of challenge in any family. Siobhan now has a caring partner who is in employment. This new partner has also been able to take on some parenting responsibility for Poppy, even though he agrees with Siobhan that Poppy's behaviour is rather unpredictable and challenging. Both parents clearly adore the boys.

Poppy's health records show that there was repeated contact with universal and specialist services in her first few years of life, with referrals made to a primary mental health worker, a family centre and Home-Start.[1] There were also reports of frequent temper tantrums and destructive behaviour, which had been observed by a number of professionals who visited, including the health visitor. Those who had contact with Poppy in the pre-school years were sympathetic to the difficulties her mother faced, but as well as witnessing the negative behaviour, they were also often greeted with smiles and demands for a cuddle. Although professionals felt uncomfortable about admitting that there was little more that could be offered, they could not help but agree that Poppy was, in her mother's words, 'a devil of a child'.

In order to provide some respite from the difficulties that she presented to her mother, Poppy was able to access a funded placement at nursery just before her third birthday. However, her attendance was poor and she required considerable support in gaining the confidence to play with the other children. On a more positive note, the nursery staff reported that Poppy was a child who sought to please, however, they added that she was rather quiet and attributed this to a delay in her speech development. A referral for Poppy to be seen by a speech and language therapist had been made by the health visitor, but after she was not taken to two appointments her name was removed from the waiting list.

[1]See www.home-start.org.uk/homepage.

Practice point

Over-friendliness with strangers and attention-seeking behaviour in young children may indicate a problematic attachment. An insecure attachment can be a feature of emotional abuse and other forms of child maltreatment (NCCWCH 2009).

Domestic violence and abuse

Children who are affected by domestic violence and abuse (DVA) may suffer from a range of health, developmental and behavioural difficulties. The evidence to link DVA and child maltreatment is well established. The high prevalence of DVA is concerning, and as Radford *et al.* (2011) found, nearly one-quarter of 18–24-year-olds in their study had experienced the effects of DVA in their childhoods. Such children may have frequent moves and will suffer the loss of their home, room, possessions, friends and school. Adolescents may begin to distance themselves and are at a greater risk of running away and engaging in anti-social or criminal behaviour. Although victims will try to protect their children, the ability to parent well is compromised, and the mother–child relationship may break down. Early help and support can help to minimize harm and may reduce the likelihood of child victims perpetrating DVA in adulthood (NICE 2014a). An extremely useful toolkit developed by the Department of Health provides a comprehensive over-view of the effects of DVA on children of various ages, and also notes factors that improve a child's resilience (DH 2009). While women are the main victims of DVA, it can affect men, trans-people and those in same sex relationships.

Case 1 continued

Poppy is now at primary school and is in Year 1. Her teachers assess that she is a bright child, who is not reaching her potential. She is often unhappy and appears to have difficulties in making friends, in part because she has a tendency to be spiteful. Following a discussion at a parent–teacher evening, where concerns about Poppy's behaviour were once again raised, Siobhan takes Poppy to the GP and a referral is made to CAMHS. Joe, who is a mental health nurse, and has specialized in CAMHS, sees Poppy and her mother at a tier-two clinic (see below for an explanation of the CAMHS four-tier strategic frame-work). A provisional diagnosis of oppositional defiant disorder (ODD) is made.

CAMHS four-tier strategic framework

The CAMHS four-tier strategic framework is a widely accepted conceptual framework for the commissioning, planning and delivery of services to children and young people who are experiencing mental health difficulties.

Tier one services are delivered by practitioners who are not mental health specialists, such as health visitors, school nurses and GPs. They will promote good mental health, offer general advice and treatment for less severe problems and refer to more specialist services where necessary. An example would be intervention offered in a case of mild anxiety that is beginning to affect everyday functioning and well-being.

Tier two services are offered by CAMHS specialists, such as primary mental health workers, psychologists and counsellors working in community and primary care settings. They will offer consultation to families and other practitioners, outreach to identify severe or complex needs and training to non-specialist practitioners working at tier one. An example would be intervention in conduct disorders.

Tier three services are usually provided by a multi-disciplinary team working in a community mental health clinic or child psychiatry outpatient department. The team will provide more specialized care for children, young people and their families with more severe, complex or persistent disorders such as obsessive-compulsive rituals.

Tier four comprises highly specialist, often regionally based services for children and young people with the most serious mental health difficulties. Care may be provided by outpatient teams or within inpatient facilities. These may include forensic adolescent units, eating disorder units, specialist neuro-psychiatric units and intensive care. An example of tier-four care would be for a young person at high risk of serious self-harm.

Note: CAMHS inpatient care includes young people up to the age of 18 years. If an under-16-year-old is admitted to an adult mental health unit then this should be reported to specialist commissioners as a 'serious incident'. Data are also collected on 16- and 17-year-olds who are admitted as a 'reportable incident'.

Oppositional defiant disorder

'Oppositional defiant disorder' (ODD) is a term used to describe disruptive and aggressive behaviour in the home that goes beyond that which may be considered 'normal' in childhood. While it can be linked to those who have a difficult temperament, attention deficit hyperactive disorder (ADHD) or learning difficulties, it can also present as a result of negative parenting styles, bullying and abuse (Royal College of Psychiatrists 2012). Treatment can take a variety of forms, including parenting programmes, individual or family psychotherapy and cognitive behavioural therapy (CBT). In some cases, particularly as a first line of provision, input from a primary mental health worker can be helpful.

Case 1 continued

Working very closely with Siobhan, Poppy and her stepfather, Joe, the CAMHS practitioner, devises a programme of tailored therapy that includes a focus on positive parenting techniques. These will not only be helpful to Poppy, but also serve as a useful adjunct to ensure that the twins are parented in a way that will promote good mental health for the future. Joe liaises with the family health visitor, GP and the school. His review of the records reflects his concerns that Poppy was somewhat of a scapegoat for her mother's difficulties surrounding the violent and destructive relationship with Poppy's father. He is also concerned that previous professionals have demonstrated sympathy and support for Siobhan with her relationship, housing and financial problems and her 'difficult child' and failed to respond to the fact that this mother had frequently sought to express a real difficulty in loving a child who resulted from a brutal relationship with the father. Joe judges there to be early evidence of an emotionally abusive relationship between parent and child and that this has contributed to the development of her conduct disorder. Siobhan has been unable to develop a responsive and protective relationship with her daughter. Furthermore, it is concerning that this mother has expressed negativity in the presence of professionals who floundered in their ability to offer a helpful response. In summary, Joe feels that there is past evidence of emotional abuse and a failure by professionals to consider the best interests of the child. He discusses these concerns with his supervisor.

 Child's perspective

Poppy is a victim of emotional abuse. In the first three years of her life she witnessed (through seeing, sensing and hearing) the violent and abusive relationship between her parents and was frightened, confused and distressed. Parenting has lacked warmth, boundaries and, above all, consistency. Her mother, because of her own difficulties, has often been emotionally flat, neglectful and unpredictable in responding to her daughter's needs. The arrival of younger siblings has intensified Poppy's feelings of rejection. She craves attention, but lacks trust and self-worth, and uses negative behaviour to ensure that she is noticed. Lots of people have visited the house to talk to her mother and stepfather. Very few of them have spoken to her.

Markers of good practice: the role of the health care team

The case of Poppy demonstrates what can happen when professionals are drawn to the (very real) problems of parents and lose sight of the best interests of the child.

Poppy was born in very difficult circumstances and by her own admission Siobhan felt that she was a 'difficult child to love'. Early input from the health visitor and others should have ensured that additional support and advice was aimed at developing mother–child attachment through a more positive and child-centred approach.

Joe appears to be the first professional who has focused on the meaning of the parental difficulties for the child and the impact of an emotionally abusive relationship on the development of ODD. More attention should have been given to the fact that the nursery did not witness the degree of challenging behaviour that was reported to be happening at home, as well as the reported 'over-friendliness' with strangers.

Joe completes clear, contemporaneous records of the events and his actions (NMC 2015). He also follows local clinical supervision policy in recording the outcomes and actions from his deliberations with his supervisor.

There will be a need to review the situation and consider whether any current concerns, or failure to respond to treatment, should lead to a referral to children's social care.

Case 2: Tyra – a 'little mother' to her siblings

Tyra is 13 years old and in Year 9 at school. She has three younger siblings, the youngest of whom is 22 months old. Lately Tyra has been either missing school, or arriving late looking somewhat tired and distracted. Her school work is suffering. Teachers are concerned that she will slip further behind with her studies at a time when she should be focusing her thoughts on her GCSE choices for the following year. They discuss their concerns that all is not well at home with the school nurse and the education welfare officer.

A decision is made that, in the first instance, Tyra should be persuaded to see the school nurse at the lunchtime drop in session; if there is little visible improvement in attendance and demeanour then the educational welfare officer will pick up the case. When the school nurse meets Tyra, she is noticeably pale and quiet. Eventually it transpires that she has been providing care for her younger siblings, including managing shopping on a very limited budget, preparing meals and feeding and bathing the toddler. She has also been taking the middle two children to their primary school most days. The school is located about half a mile from her secondary school. At the weekends Tyra has been cleaning and washing clothes. She has not been seeing her friends lately. Tyra's overriding concerns are for her parents, Tracy and Dave, who have been staying in bed and are sometimes angry or difficult to rouse. Despite trying to keep on top of things, Tyra is very ashamed of the state of the house and is worried about the increasingly clingy behaviour of her toddler brother. Tyra's parents are known to have problems with alcohol, and are also thought to have used heroin and benzodiazepines in the past. The local substance misuse service has previously been involved with the family and the GP will re-refer, as appropriate, after consulting the parents. Tyra is extremely cautious about sharing her story, expressing a wish for the family to stay together and for things to be 'like they used to be'. Tyra is effectively a 'young carer' whose needs for a safe and secure childhood in which she can achieve her full potential are not being met. All of the children are at risk of suffering from neglect and emotional abuse. After seeking support from her manager, and discussing her concerns for the children's well-being at a home visit to the parents, the school nurse makes a child protection referral to children's social care services.

Young carers

Working Together (HM Government 2015a) has firmly placed the particular needs of young carers within the framework for safeguarding and child protection. This reflects new legislation within the Children and Families Act 2014 that require local authorities to ensure that the right support and services are in place for families with caring needs. Although a perception of young carers normally reflects those children and young people caring for a parent with a physical illness or disability, parents who are chronic substance misusers may place unreasonable demands on their older children that include domestic tasks and the care of younger siblings.

Parental substance misuse

The risks to children from parental substance misuse are present from conception to adulthood. These risks include foetal alcohol syndrome, the distress from withdrawal seen in neonates, the impact on families' finances, risks to children's safety and the neglectful parenting that sits alongside parents' preoccupation with their own needs (Davies and Ward 2012). Substance misuse is a known risk factor for child maltreatment (HM Government 2015a) and a contributory factor in child maltreatment deaths and serious incidents. Parental substance misuse was recorded in nearly half (42 per cent) of the 184 serious case reviews analysed by Brandon *et al.* (2012). For many substance misusing parents, drugs or alcohol are one part of a multiplicity of problems that include mental health difficulties, family relationship breakdown, isolation and poor socioeconomic circumstances.

According to figures highlighted in guidance for schools on supporting pupils of parents who have substance misuse difficulties, there are thought to be as many as 335,000 children in the UK living with parental drug dependency and more than a million living with problematic parental alcohol use (Princess Royal Trust for Carers/Children's Society 2010). As the guidance notes, these children and young people are often engaged in providing physical care and emotional support to their parents, as well as coping with household chores and the care of siblings. It adds that these young carers can find it very difficult to seek help from agencies because they are concerned about the stigma of parental substance misuse, a feeling of betrayal of their parents and the impact of any likely intervention on their family life. The guidance also acknowledges the dangers and risks faced by children and young people within the context of parental substance misuse (e.g. from drug paraphernalia, others visiting the household or the increased likelihood of becoming users themselves) and calls for school nurses to be available to support affected pupils' health and well-being and to undertake home visits to their families. The links to safeguarding and child protection are acknowledged.

Although a great deal has been achieved in terms of better recognition and response to the issues raised by problematic parental substance misuse in recent years, it is still seen as an area where improvements can be made. The seminal report *Hidden Harm*, which was published in 2003 following an inquiry by the Advisory Council on the Misuse of Drugs (ACMD), raised awareness of the extent of the problem and sought to ensure a timely and appropriate response to meet the needs of families. The report contained a number of recommendations, some of which were specifically aimed at early years, schools and health services, including those dealing specifically with drug and alcohol problems with adults who may be parents or carers. The over-arching messages from the work included the recognition of the serious risk of harm to children of all ages and the benefits to children of early help and successful treatment of parental substance misuse problems. *Hidden Harm* recognized that by working together services can take many practical steps to protect and improve the health and well-being of affected children and young people. Two of the *Hidden Harm* recommendations were aimed specifically at substance misuse services:

- Drug and alcohol agencies should recognize that they have a responsibility towards the dependent children of their clients and aim to provide accessible and effective support for parents and their children, either directly or through good links with other relevant services.
- The training of staff in drug and alcohol agencies should include a specific focus on learning how to assess and meet the needs of clients as parents and their children.

(ACMD 2003:17).

Evidence put forward in a continuing strategy to address the harmful effects of parental substance misuse suggests that children's and adults' services are improving in the ways in which they are working together as part of a wider 'team around the family' (HM Government 2012). This improvement reflects the input of nurses and midwives from both services as well as that of other key players.

An Early Help Assessment (EHA) (see Chapter 2) and a joined-up approach between child health and substance misuse services in working with substance misusing parents to identify the risks, and also the protective factors for their children, can help to minimize harm and prevent an escalation to child protection referral. However, where there is a lack of parental consent, compliance or concordance with an EHA plan or treatment regime (and disguised compliance is not uncommon in this client group) and/or evidence that children are at risk of, or suffering from, child maltreatment, then a referral to children's social care for more in-depth assessment and enquiries will be needed (as in the case presented here).

Case 2 continued

Fred, a mental health nurse by background, is a member of the multidisciplinary substance misuse community team which provides tier-three[2] services including stabilization, detoxification and counselling in cases of complex substance misuse and dependency. He has been allocated as the key worker for Dave and Tracy. Fred's care plan identifies the needs of the parents, Tyra and her siblings and aims to do the following:

* stabilize, and then reduce, the parents' substance misuse, working towards detoxification and abstinence;
* liaise with the health visitor and school nurse to ensure that the children's health needs are met;
* support the parents to ensure that their eldest three children are attending school.

In addition, Fred will liaise with children's social care. His role here is to provide support and advice to children's social care in planning to best meet the needs of the children. Because of the intense nature of his input, he may also be the first professional to recognize any deterioration in parenting or additional concerns about the well-being of the children. It is likely that social care will consider these children as being at risk of emotional abuse and also of neglect. If a decision is made to proceed to child protection enquiries, then Fred will contribute to these together with other colleagues from health services. However, his contribution, and that of children's social care, will not replace the input of core universal services.

The initial child protection conference

In the case of Tyra and her siblings, continuing concerns from the school nurse, health visitor, GP, substance misuse and educational services about

---

[2]Like CAMHS, substance misuse services are provided within a four-tier framework.

the behaviours of the parents and the welfare of the children are such that a strategy discussion is held and a decision made to initiate Children Act 1989 'Section 47' (i.e. child protection) enquiries.

As a key professional providing care to parents who are experiencing substance misuse problems, Fred engages with the statutory child protection processes (HM Government 2015a) by providing information on the parents' treatment programmes, their concordance with the treatment and the functional impact of their addiction. He discusses the information that he will be disclosing with the family, the rationale for sharing, and seeks their consent to do so.

Enquiries under Section 47 of the Children Act 1989

Section 47 sets out the duties of the local authority (i.e. children's social care services) in making enquiries to decide whether compulsory intervention is needed to safeguard or promote the welfare of a child. It also places agencies, such as health services, under a duty to assist the local authority in carrying out such enquiries.

The local authority children's social care department has the lead responsibility for undertaking child protection enquiries. A social worker will begin an assessment of the children's needs. The assessment will be systematic, dynamic and informed by a local protocol that has been drawn up to reflect the evidence for best practice. It will be a continuing process that will be centred on the child and focused on action and outcomes. The framework for assessment normally reflects the three domains that also inform EHA – i.e. the child's developmental needs, parenting capacity and family and environmental factors – but will be more in depth. Diversity will be respected. The child and their family will be fully involved in the assessment process and the child will be spoken to alone. Obtaining children and young people's views and wishes is crucial to the assessment process and it is important that they have an opportunity to be seen both with, and without, their parents or carers. In gathering information to inform the assessment, the social worker has a responsibility to liaise with other services involved with the family and to seek their views. This will include universal services (midwives, health visitors, school nurses) as well as any specialist health service provision.

Initial child protection conferences (ICPCs) are normally held within 15 working days of a strategy discussion's decision to initiate Section 47 enquiries. This is an opportunity to bring together family members, the child (where appropriate) and the professionals who are most involved with the child and family. The purpose of an ICPC is to:

- bring together and analyse the information that has been obtained in relation to the child's health and developmental needs and the parents' ability to meet these needs within the context of the family and environment;

- make a judgement on the harm suffered by the child and the likelihood of the child suffering significant harm in the future; and
- decide what future action will be needed to safeguard and promote the welfare of the child in the future, including whether the child should be made the subject of a child protection plan.

ICPCs can be very large gatherings and this carries with it the risk that the children and families who are the subject of the conference may feel intimidated. An ICPC will typically involve the following:

- the child, if they are of an appropriate age/understanding;
- family members (parents and sometimes extended family such as grandparents);
- advocates for the child or family;
- a conference chair;
- children's social care staff, including the lead social worker who has undertaken the assessment;
- professionals involved with the children (e.g. midwife, health visitor or school nurse, CAMHS practitioner, GP, early years or teaching staff, paediatrician);
- professionals involved with the parents (e.g. mental health or substance misuse practitioners, GP);
- those involved in the investigations (e.g. the police);
- local authority legal services (child care).

The role of the conference chair

Formal child protection conferences are highly likely to be stressful for children, young people and their families due to the nature of the concerns and the professional scrutiny of parenting and family life. There is frequently sociocultural diversity between professionals and the family. The conference chair, who will be accountable to the director of children's services, but independent to operational or line management responsibilities for the family, will meet the child and parents before the conference to ensure that they understand the purpose and process of the meeting.

The nursing contribution

Nurses, midwives and health visitors who are invited to attend an ICPC will be expected to bring details of their involvement with the child and family to the conference. This will be in the form of written reports that will include details of involvement with the family, and a chronology of significant events. These should be prepared to reflect, as far as possible, the domains for assessment and include practitioners' knowledge of the child's developmental needs and the capacity of the parents to meet those needs within their family and environmental context (DH 2015). A good quality report will include an analysis that reflects both strengths and difficulties within the domains. Resilience and protective factors should be considered in balance with the level of vulnerability and risk. In providing information to an ICPC it is important to be able to distinguish between fact, observation, allegation and opinion. Information may be provided from another source, but this should be made clear.

A report from a health visitor, for example, may include:

• name, qualifications and employer, how long employed in current post and how long family have been known to the practitioner;

• demographic details of the family including who is in the household and names and relationships of significant others;

• brief chronology of health-visiting contacts with the family (e.g. core universal programme or targeted programme, dates of contacts, assessment of parental engagement and compliance);

• details of child's (or children's) health and developmental needs, including their presentation and demeanour, any specific health problems and unmet needs (physical, social and emotional);

• an assessment of the parental capacity to meet the health and developmental needs of the child (or children), including an assessment of capacity to change;

• details of the wider family and environment, including housing and social integration;

• an analysis of the future safety, health and developmental needs of the child or children, and how these may be met.

Child protection case conference reports should be shared with the family in advance of the conference. It is also usual practice for the report to be shared with, or signed off by, a manager or safeguarding lead prior to the conference.

The form and function of the initial child protection conference

As noted above, the ICPC can be a large gathering of family members and professionals. Although the length of time a conference takes will be dependent on the complexity of the case, as well as the number of children in the family, proceedings normally take about two hours. Under the direction of the conference chair, and following a round of introductions, those attending an ICPC will begin by sharing their reports (with the social worker normally giving their report and outlining the concerns at the outset). The information gathered will build and present a rich tapestry of the daily lived experiences of the child or young person and help to inform the actions and decisions of the conference. Parents (and, where age appropriate, the child or young person) will be able to respond to concerns raised and the chair will ensure that opportunities are made available to clarify any points of uncertainty or challenge.

After hearing from the family and professionals, the conference chair will seek to sum up the child protection concerns that have been expressed and invite agency representatives to express an opinion as to whether or not there is a need for a statutory child protection plan. This will then be enacted on the basis of a majority decision that the child has suffered, or is likely to suffer, significant harm, and is, or remains, at risk of suffering significant harm in the future. The chair will also direct the conference in determining which category of abuse or neglect will be recorded (in some cases more than one category is given, although the use of multiple categories for child protection plans has been declining). Where there is more than one child in a family, a separate discussion will take place for each child.

Tyra and her siblings: subject to a child protection plan

In the case of Tyra and her siblings, concerns shared at the ICPC were such that a decision was made that Tyra would be made subject to a child protection plan under the category of 'emotional abuse'. This reflects the fact that Tyra's caring responsibilities for her siblings were interfering with her school attendance and other normal daily activities (NCCWCH 2009). The conference chair concluded the decision-making by reflecting the fact that there were 'age or developmentally inappropriate expectations being imposed on [her]' (HM Government 2015a:92). In addition, Tyra's siblings were made subject to a plan because they were considered to be at risk of neglect. The health visitor, the school nurse and the substance misuse nurse will all have a part to play in the core group of professionals and family members that will develop and implement the plan. At the end of the ICPC dates were set for a core group meeting and the first review child protection conference (RCPC) (see Chapter 7).

 Child's perspective

Tyra loves her parents and siblings very much, but is worried and embarrassed about her parents' substance misuse. She has tried to manage to look after everyone, but is anxious about missing school. She would love to have her friends round for a 'sleep-over' but she is ashamed of the state of her house and knows that her younger siblings will want to join in, too.

Markers of good practice: the role of the substance misuse nurse

Fred acknowledges that he has a role in the assessment of the needs of any children where there is parental substance misuse. He is particularly concerned to ensure that Tyra is able to attend school and take part in activities with her peer group – i.e. to ensure that there are no 'age or developmentally inappropriate expectations being imposed upon [her]' that are indicative of emotional abuse (HM Government 2015a:92).

Tyra is provided with preventative advice and support in relation to the increased potential for her to become a user. Ensuring that she achieves her potential at school and is able to maintain a friendship group are important factors in achieving self-esteem and resilience.

Fred completes a care plan that includes the steps to be taken to ensure the needs of the children are met and liaises with universal health services (GP, health visitor and school nurse). He seeks consent from Dave and Tracy to share information appropriately in line with information-sharing guidelines (HM Government 2015b).

Fred monitors the well-being of the children from his perspective of the impact of parental substance misuse on the ability to provide good enough parenting and liaises with children's social care accordingly. He seeks advice from his safeguarding leads (named professionals) where necessary.

Fred attends the strategy discussion and the ICPC, for which he produces a report. The report outlines his care plans for the family and the engagement of Dave and Tracy in their treatment regimes, and includes an analysis of strengths and difficulties. The report is shared with the family prior to the conference.

Fred completes clear, contemporaneous records of the events and his actions (NMC 2015). He also follows local clinical supervision policy in recording the outcomes and actions from his deliberations with his supervisor.

Case 3: Nilay – a hidden child

Nilay is 9 years old and has cerebral palsy with associated spastic quadriplegia and communication difficulties. He is the third child of Asha and Taj, and was born overseas at 29 weeks' gestation following a difficult pregnancy. Nilay's disability means that he requires a high level of care to meet his basic needs; however, his parents have been reluctant to allow professionals into the home and have been largely managing the care themselves, with some additional help from extended family. Nilay has recently been unwell with a series of chest infections and is becoming increasingly frail. Following a routine paediatric review a decision was made for Nilay to have a percutaneous endoscopic gastrostomy (PEG) feeding tube to provide enteral nutrition support, with the anticipation that an increased intake of calories and protein would improve his physical well-being and help to prevent infection.

Vicky, a children's community nurse, calls to see Nilay and his family at home to support the management of his new feeding regime. On entering the home, Vicky is greeted by Nilay's parents and elder sisters and taken to the living room where she is surprised to see little evidence of the equipment usually associated with children with similar needs. Nilay, it transpires, is in his room, being a ground floor annexe at the back of the main house. A grandmother sleeps in an adjacent room.

As this is her first visit to the family, Vicky undertakes a detailed holistic assessment to support her care planning. She considers the need for an interpreter to support her communication with Nilay and his parents, but finds that Taj is able to translate for his wife, where needed. Vicky discovers that while Nilay appears to be reasonably well cared for physically, he is not currently receiving any formal education. His parents report that they felt that there was no suitable provision and lay claim to providing some input themselves. Vicky's overriding concern is that Nilay is somewhat hidden from others. She discusses her unease with her manager, as she is worried that Nilay's isolation and apparent lack of interaction with other children, including somewhat limited contact with his siblings, may be affecting his opportunities to reach his potential, albeit that this is limited by his special needs. This state of affairs has been recognized in a study undertaken by Robert and Harris (2002) who found that immigrants and asylum-seeking families had a greater fear of being seen as 'doubly' different where family members were disabled.

Multiple challenges

The challenges for professionals in this case are numerous. As we discuss in the following chapter, children with a learning or physical disability are at greater risk of child maltreatment, but less likely to have concerns about possible harm raised (Murray and Osborne 2009). Nilay's parents and family appear devoted, however, as the statutory definition notes: 'overprotection and limitation of exploration and learning, or preventing the child participating in normal social interaction' is indicative of emotional abuse (HM Government 2015a:93).

In addition to the challenges provided by this complex case, it is my experience that children's community nurses do not necessarily have the same traditions of safeguarding and child protection skills and awareness as, for example, health visitors and school nurses. This may be due in part to a lack of appropriate learning opportunities and access to named professionals and others for specialist supervision. However, anecdotally, I have witnessed a tendency for these practitioners to develop very close relationships with parents and carers, who themselves are often struggling with the physical, emotional and financial burdens of caring for a child with complex needs; a finding that was in common with an inspection report on the protection of disabled children (Ofsted 2012). This state of affairs can lead to a failure by children's community nurses to consider the daily lived experience of the child (Laming 2009). Thus, Vicky is likely to need a high degree of support and access to good 'child protection' oriented supervision to allow her to advocate for Nilay and to ensure that he is given the maximum opportunity to develop his potential. Importantly, her skills in child-centred assessment have enabled her to identify that his needs are currently not being met.

Nilay: next steps

With the support of her manager and the named nurse safeguarding children, Vicky arranges a professional network meeting to share her concerns about Nilay's isolation and educational needs. Those in the children's disability team attend. The team is already aware of the fact that Nilay has become physically frail. However, it transpires that, with the exception of a paediatric occupational therapist who has undertaken home visits to assist and advise on home adaptations, Nilay has generally been seen in a community clinic or hospital setting. Therefore the concerns about his apparent seclusion and the impact that this may have on his emotional well-being have not been identified previously. In addition, there is also a possibility that the cultural diversity of the family (including language differences) has proved to be a barrier and that their status as newly arrived immigrants has prevented them from claiming Disability Living Allowance at the current time.

Through his isolation, Nilay is missing out on normal childhood opportunities for play, education and friendship. This contravenes the UNCRC, Children Act 1989 and the provisions of the Equality Act 2010. The social worker for children with disabilities is asked to liaise with child protection colleagues in social care to consider an assessment of Nilay's health and developmental needs in line with Section 17, Children Act 1989 and to identify the best way forward in working with his family to ensure that these are met. A specialist interpreter will be part of the team to ensure that Nilay's voice is heard. His educational needs will be assessed under the provisions for children with disabilities and an education and health care plan (EHC) drawn up (DfE/DH 2014). In addition, arrangements will be made to ensure that Nilay has access to short breaks, to allow the family respite from his care needs and quality time with his siblings.

Child's perspective

Due to his communication difficulties, Nilay finds it difficult to have his needs met. He is often unwell with chest infections and in pain from his condition. He feels isolated and lonely. Nilay is dependent on the care from his family, yet will need the intervention of professionals to make his daily lived experiences as positive and productive as possible in what will inevitably be a shortened lifespan.

Markers of good practice: the role of the children's community nurse

In her provision of care, Vicky demonstrates sensitivity to differing family structures and lifestyles and an understanding that child-rearing patterns can vary across different racial, ethnic and cultural groups. However, her ability to consider the child's perspective means that she is unable to condone the family's approach to his care.

Vicky seeks supervision from her manager and initiates a professional network meeting to share her concerns and to consider next actions.

Vicky completes clear, contemporaneous records of the events and her actions (NMC 2015).

Summary

This chapter has considered emotional abuse in childhood. As noted at the outset, emotional abuse is present in all forms of child maltreatment, but may occur on its own. The statutory definition of emotional abuse describes a range of situations of concern, but it may be best summarized as 'a relationship rather than an event'. Thus this form of abuse will most typically involve difficulties in the parent–child relationship. The three scenarios outlined in this chapter describe emotional abuse in the context of an unloved child who develops a conduct disorder, an adolescent who takes responsibility for the care of her parents and siblings and a disabled child whose developmental needs are compromised by a lack of opportunity for education and social interaction with his peers. The nursing staff involved in these fictitious cases included a CAMHS practitioner, a substance misuse nurse and a community children's nurse. The unifying feature in terms of taking action to safeguard and promote the welfare of these children was the ability of these professionals to consider the 'daily lived experience' of the child.

Key points

- Nurses and midwives who see children in the course of their practice should be familiar with child care and development and have a sound understanding of indicators of possible child maltreatment.

- An understanding of the needs of children and the features of good parenting is helpful in the prevention, early identification of and response to emotional abuse.

- Assessments of children in need consider the child's developmental factors, family and environmental factors and parenting capacity.

- Sensitivity to race, culture and ethnicity is important, however, child abuse cannot be condoned for religious or cultural reasons.

- Child protection conferences should consider strengths and protective factors, as well as risks.

5

Child sexual abuse

Learning outcomes

This chapter will help you to:

- Understand the features of sexual abuse as a form of child maltreatment.
- Be able to identify indicators and behaviours that may be associated with sexual abuse in the course of your practice.
- Develop your understanding of the increased risk of child maltreatment for children and young people with disabilities.
- Make a professional contribution to a child protection plan.
- Know how to respond to a disclosure of adult behaviour that is indicative of child sexual abuse.

Introduction

This chapter considers child sexual abuse and begins by outlining the defining attributes of this form of maltreatment and the possible presenting indicators. Following the format of the previous chapters, three fictitious scenarios, which are based on the reality of practice in cases of child sexual abuse, are presented. As before, these practical examples cannot be fully inclusive of the range of behaviours and features of this form of abuse, but are intended to trigger the development of knowledge and understanding that will help nurses and midwives to be confident and competent in recognizing and responding to child maltreatment.

- Case 1: Maryam, aged 14 years, is attending a young persons' contraception and sexual health clinic with a friend. She is seeking a pregnancy test.
- Case 2: Jodie, a 10-year-old with progressive learning disabilities, has begun attending a respite care facility provided by the local children's hospice. She and her family are supported by Marcus, a registered nurse (learning disability), who provides an outreach service from the hospice.
- Case 3: Stewart, who is an adult mental health service client, discloses that he has been accessing indecent images of children on the internet.

Building on the knowledge and understanding that you have gained about the pathway for child protection referral, the strategy discussion, the Children Act 1989 Section 47 (child protection enquiries) and the ICPC, this chapter introduces the child protection plan. The plan, which follows the initial child protection conference consensus decision that a child or young person may be at continuing risk of significant harm, informs the process by which agencies work together with children, young people and their families to ensure their future safety and protection. Nurses and midwives from both universal and specialist services may have a key role in leading, or supporting, actions that are outlined in the plan. We begin by defining child sexual abuse.

Child sexual abuse

The *Working Together* definition of child sexual abuse is as follows:

> [Sexual abuse] involves forcing or enticing a child or young person to take part in sexual activities, not necessarily involving a high level of violence, whether or not the child is aware of what is happening. The activities may involve physical contact, including assault by penetration (for example, rape or oral sex) or non-penetrative acts such as masturbation, kissing, rubbing and touching outside of clothing. They may also include non-contact activities, such as involving children looking at, or in the production of, sexual images, watching sexual activities, encouraging children to behave in sexually inappropriate ways, or grooming a child in preparation for abuse (including via the internet). Sexual abuse is not solely perpetrated by adult males. Women can also commit acts of sexual abuse, as can other children.
>
> (HM Government 2015a:93)

Polnay *et al.* (2007) note that the notion of child sexual abuse being part of the spectrum of mainstream child maltreatment occurred some 20 years after child physical abuse was first highlighted to health professionals. This was, they add, in spite of the fact that sexual abuse had been raised as a possible form of harm in childhood many years previously by pioneers such as Freud. Society's acceptance of the existence of this form of maltreatment has seemingly lagged behind that of professionals, although there are signs that the 'celebrity' sexual abuse cases (see Chapter 1) have resulted in a greater awareness and willingness to acknowledge and report it, even if the abuse happened several decades previously. However, there is evidence that sufferers today may still experience difficulty in telling their story, and ultimately receiving the care and protection that they need (Allnock and Miller 2013). Such difficulties can be compounded by the fact that the sexually abused child may be unaware that what they are experiencing is abusive, in part, because they may have been 'groomed' by their perpetrator and also because of their age and developmental status.

Quotes from adult survivors of child sexual abuse

'Why do I feel so bad, like it was my fault? I didn't know what was happening to me at the time. I didn't even know what sex was . . .'

'He used to say to me that this was our secret and I should never tell anyone, especially mum and dad (I didn't).'

'When I was thirteen, I suddenly connected what he was doing to me with playground dirty jokes . . .'

'If I had had someone to talk to that I could trust, I may have opened up but my problem was that I was full of fear and could not bring myself to talk to someone . . .'

(National Commission of Inquiry into the
Prevention of Child Abuse 1996:170–2)

The number of children and young people who are made subject to a child protection plan because they are at risk of, or suffering from, sexual abuse is low, with approximately 4.5 per cent of plans being made within this category of abuse. However, a recently published evidence appraisal of intra-familial child sexual abuse reflects the belief that such figures do not bear witness to the reported prevalence of this form of maltreatment (Horvath et al. 2014). The study by Radford et al. (2011), highlighted in previous chapters, is particularly helpful in determining the statistics for child sexual abuse. This is because it draws on the experiences of children and young adults from across the population, rather than simply those who come to the attention of statutory child protection agencies. In terms of both contact and non-contact sexual abuse by adults, or peers, across childhood, Radford et al. found reported rates of 1.2 per cent for under 11-year-olds, 16.5 per cent for those aged 11–17 years and 24.1 per cent for those aged 18–24 years. Co-existence with physical violence and other forms of maltreatment was a notable feature in many of the cases. Child sexual abuse was reported to occur most often within the context of the family or was perpetrated by those known to the children and young people. Girls were more often victims and males more often perpetrators. Two-thirds of the reported abuse was perpetrated by a peer.

Perpetrators and victims of child sexual abuse are drawn from across the social spectrum. However, certain groups of children are noted to be at greater risk of harm. These groups include disabled children (Murray and Osborne 2009), children in care and those whose parents are experiencing adult mental health or substance misuse problems (Nelson 2009). Perpetrators of intra-familial child sexual abuse may have their own history of childhood abuse, dysfunctional backgrounds, disordered attachment and problems with intimate relationships (Horvath et al. 2014). This evidence has important implications for health professionals, as the high-risk groups are likely to be accessing a range of services. This means that many nurses and midwives are in a position to recognize and respond to children and young people at risk of sexual abuse, or those adults who pose such a risk. Nevertheless, it is also important to be aware of the difficulties that children and young people have in disclosing sexual maltreatment. For example, many of Allnock and Miller's (2013) sample of child sexual abuse victims reported numerous attempts to disclose to a family member, friend or person in authority (e.g. a teacher). Furthermore, the disclosures were, on average, 7.8 years after the abuse, and the younger the child the longer the delay. Of those that did disclose, many had an unhelpful response that added to their negative experiences. Less than one-third of mothers reportedly took any action following the disclosure, with some actively minimizing events or disbelieving their child. Nelson (2009:24) summarizes the reasons for non-disclosure of childhood sexual abuse as 'deep shame, self-blame, fear of other children's rejection, fear of retaliation and the expectation of being disbelieved'.

These are fundamental issues for nurses and midwives. An acknowledgement of the existence and prevalence of child sexual abuse, and the difficulties that victims encounter in disclosing their experiences, are key factors in offering a helpful and therapeutic response. The stories of 'victim-survivors' (Allnock and Miller 2013) reflect numerous missed opportunities for intervention and support.

Practice question

Nelson (2009) suggests that for a worried young person or adult to confide abuse within a health care setting professionals need to:

- be welcoming;
- create an atmosphere of respect;
- be receptive to the possibility of child sexual abuse;
- be sensitive; and
- offer open-minded, non-judgemental listening.

How can this be assured in your area of practice?

Indicators of child sexual abuse

Drawing on the evidence-based guidelines published by the RCPCH,[1] the NCCWCH guidelines (2009:47) conclude that observable signs of child sexual abuse are 'relatively uncommon'. The guidelines attribute this finding to the

---

[1]The guidance has been updated and was published in May 2015.

timing of the examination relative to the abuse and the difficulties of conducting comparative studies in this area. Sexual abuse does not usually leave lasting traces and damage to the anogenital area is reported to heal quickly (De Laar and Lagro-Janssen 2009). However, it is important to note that children and young people presenting with suspected contact child sexual abuse should be assessed by those with specialist expertise and access to a colposcope. Where possible, these children and young people should be given a choice as to the gender of their examiner and be supported by a non-abusing parent, or other adult of their choice, if they so wish. Repeated examinations of this intimate nature may be viewed as being abusive in themselves. In my experience, nurses and midwives have had to intervene to advocate for protecting the child from an inexperienced, but concerned, clinician who is keen to make a 'diagnosis'. An exception to this state of affairs would be in the rare cases where urgent medical attention may be required.

Anogenital signs and symptoms that are suggestive of child sexual abuse include bruising, laceration, swelling or abrasion in the absence of a suitable explanation, persistent soreness and bleeding or discharge without medical explanation and with associated behavioural or emotional change. The guidelines tackle the controversial issue of the 'reflex anal dilatation' (RAD) test and conclude that this should be undertaken by an experienced professional, rather than a front-line health care practitioner (NCCWCH 2009).

Practice point

Nelson (2009) points out that people who have been sexually abused as children may be reluctant to present for health care and avoid examinations of sensitive parts of their bodies (e.g. dentistry or gynaecology). This can result in additional or preventable health problems for them and, in the case of pregnancy, unborn babies, too.

The effects of child sexual abuse

Not surprisingly, child sexual abuse can have a serious and enduring impact on the physical, emotional and sexual health of individuals across their lifespan. Horvath et al. (2014) report findings of long-term profound psychological damage, with short-term damage likely, but often hidden, due to a lack of disclosure at the time of experiencing the maltreatment.

Myers et al. (2002) provide a detailed summary of the research findings on the effects of child sexual abuse. They suggest that two decades of research into the outcomes for those who have been sexually abused as children has found a 'wide range of psychological and interpersonal problems' (p. 59). The authors link their findings to the fact that this form of abuse is frightening, painful and confusing, and that it induces shame and bewilderment.

Fundamentally, the authors propose that sexual abuse leads to responses in childhood that interfere with normal developmental processes and they summarize the effects on children and young people in terms of causing emotional distress and dysfunction, post-traumatic stress, behavioural problems, interpersonal consequences and cognitive difficulties. However, they do acknowledge that much of the research that they reviewed concerned clinical, rather than population, samples and thus may not be generalizable. Myers *et al.* also report on a number of studies that have considered the longer term outcomes for children who have been sexually abused and found that these include depression, suicidal tendencies, anxiety, poor relationships, running away from home, substance misuse, eating disorders, abnormal sexual behaviour and poor achievement at school, adding that many of these difficulties will persist into adulthood. It is thus very likely that adult survivors of sexual abuse will feature within patient and client groups in a variety of settings, including adult mental health services. Nurses and midwives thus need to be open, responsive and compassionate and know how to access additional support for this group of people (see Chapter 9).

Finally, it is worth concluding this section with a more optimistic finding on the apparently common concern that there is a high risk of those who were sexually abused as children becoming perpetrators themselves in their adult life. This is not necessarily the case (Horvath *et al.* 2014) and a consistent message for practice is that timely and responsive interventions to child sexual abuse that promote emotional and cognitive resolution may improve the chances of a positive outcome in later life.

Practice question

Given the evidence that suggests that the reactions of practitioners to a child or young person who discloses sexual abuse have an impact on the child's ability to cope, how can you ensure that you (and members of your team) are receptive, believing and responsive to the need for protection of children who have been sexually abused?

The following case scenarios describe three different presentations of child sexual abuse. Links are made to the evidence base for practice and to the statutory guidance. In each case, the actions of the nurse are described in terms of best practice.

Case 1: Maryam – a 14-year-old victim of peer abuse

Maryam, who is 14 years of age, attends a contraception and sexual health outreach clinic for young people, for a pregnancy test. She has been booked in to see Celine, the lead nurse. She is tearful and clearly anxious. Maryam has not told her family or friends that she thinks she might be pregnant. After gentle enquiry, Maryam discloses that two boys in the year above her forced her to have sex with them at a party – a party that her parents had forbidden her to attend. The boys have told her that if she tells anyone what happened they will put the pictures that they took of her semi-naked on Facebook. And in any case, given 'who she is', they tell her no one will believe her and she was 'up for it'. Every time Maryam sees the boys in the school corridors or lunch hall they nod knowingly at each other, point at their phones and laugh at her.

Practice question

How should the statutory guidance in relation to sexually active young people influence Celine's assessment of Maryam and any potential child protection needs?

Celine assesses that this may be a case of peer sexual abuse and statutory rape. Although they are only a year older than their victim, this does not appear to be consensual sex between peers. They are children, too. A response from police and children's social care is needed and a child protection medical may also be arranged. In addition to sexually assaulting her, the boys are subjecting Maryam to racially motivated intimidation and bullying (with the possibility of cyber-bullying). These boys may pose a threat to other girls. Celine will support Maryam in informing her parents about what has happened, although will not share any clinical details without her permission.

Peer sexual abuse

Based on the reports from children and young people, Radford *et al.* (2011) found that a high proportion (two-thirds) of contact sexual abuse is perpetrated by those under the age of 18 years. They note that this demonstrates a need for preventative activity, including public education and support for young people in establishing respectful relationships. In addition to their roles with individual children, school nurses can help to support teachers in the delivery of 'personal, social and health education' (PSHE).

Case 1 continued

Celine obtains as much information as possible from Maryam, and explains what she is going to share, with whom and why. After discussing the concerns with her manager, and having also sought some additional advice from her Trust's named nurse for safeguarding children, Celine makes a referral to children's social care, which will, in turn, contact the police. Information shared is proportionate and centred on protection and support. A positive pregnancy test would have additional implications. Celine offers a further appointment to provide ongoing support, and encourages Maryam to attend with her mother, for at least part of the next consultation. Given the fact that no condom was used, Celine also arranges screening for sexually transmitted infection, in line with best practice.

Practice point

Concerns about confidentiality are frequently cited as a reason that prevents young people from accessing contraception and sexual health advice and treatment. If information has to be shared, it is important to seek consent, explain why information needs to be shared, and share only what is necessary and proportionate. Decisions about information-sharing (even in cases where the decision is not to share) must always be carefully documented (HM Government 2015b).

Young person's perspective

Maryam feels fear, guilt, shame and embarrassment. She is particularly anxious about her parents' reactions to her experience and how this might result in her being ostracized from the family, especially if she is pregnant. The fact that Celine listened empathetically, believed her version of what had happened and is helping to ensure her protection from further victimization has helped to lessen her feelings of being lost and alone.

Markers of good practice: the role of the sexual health nurse

Celine recognized that Maryam was an apparent victim of peer sexual abuse; she listened to her disclosure, sought to believe her and explained what was going to happen next.

Celine informed her manager about the disclosure and sought advice and support from a safeguarding lead; she helped Maryam to think through the need to let her parents know what had happened and offered support accordingly.

Celine completes clear, contemporaneous records of the events (NMC 2015) and her actions, with particular regard to the documentation of the disclosure using Maryam's own words. Her records may contribute to any criminal justice proceedings.

Case 2: Jodie – a child with disabilities who is subject to a child protection plan

The second case study in this chapter concerns the complexities of the care of a child with a progressive disability, who is also subject to a child protection plan under the category of risk of sexual abuse. Jodie, who is 10 years of age, suffers from a rare inherited condition called Sanfilippo syndrome, one of a group of enzyme deficiency conditions known as the mucopolysaccharide diseases. Although sufferers from this group of conditions display few symptoms as babies, the disease causes progressive cellular damage and increasing levels of disability. The disease is usually described as having three phases: the first phase, in early childhood, is characterized by the onset of developmental delay (e.g. delayed speech and behavioural difficulties); the second phase, in middle childhood, is characterized by increasingly active and challenging behaviour (such as sleep disturbance and aggressive behaviour); and the third phase, from the age of about 10 years, is characterized by increasing neurological and motor difficulties, with a life expectancy of the late teens. Recently, arrangements have been made for Jodie to attend the local children's hospice for respite care. Marcus, a learning disability nurse, works within the hospice and also provides an outreach service to help to ensure joined-up care and family involvement.

Caring for a child with this condition is fraught with emotional and practical challenges. Jodie's stepfather and mother, Simon and Natasha, who have three other younger children, have recently separated following an extensive period of unhappiness. In addition to the stress caused by caring for a child with a progressive and life-limiting disability, the couple have had to come to terms with an incident involving Damian, Simon's 22-year-old son from an earlier relationship, who was suspected of sexually abusing Jodie while baby-sitting for the family. As a result of this, Jodie and her siblings are subject to a formal child protection plan because of concerns about continuing risk.

Child maltreatment and children with disabilities

There has been growing evidence that children and young people who are disabled are likely to be at a threefold greater risk of child maltreatment when compared with their non-disabled peers, yet are under-represented in safeguarding children systems. This has led to the production of a volume of supplementary guidance to *Working Together* that specifically considers the need for LSCBs and their partner agencies to address the problem and to ensure that this group of children is appropriately, and proactively, safeguarded from harm (Murray and Osborne 2009). The guidance, which is recommended reading for those involved in the care of children with disabilities and their families, specifically notes that:

> Disabled children and young people should be seen as children first. Having a disability should not and must not mask or deter an appropriate enquiry where there are child protection concerns. This premise is relevant to all

those involved with disabled children and is *particularly relevant to health care workers* given the key role they play and their close involvement with many disabled children and their families.

(Murray and Osborne 2009:13, emphasis added)

There are several possible reasons for the greater risk of maltreatment for children with disabilities. At a societal level, people with disabilities may suffer from negative attitudes, prejudice, discrimination and unequal access to goods and services. They are also more likely to suffer from bullying. The poorer outcomes for disabled children reflect reduced educational, social and recreational opportunities, an increased likelihood of poverty and social exclusion, as well as a greater chance of family breakdown and becoming a child in care. As individuals, children with disabilities may also face the challenge of speech, language and communication difficulties. Equally, those caring for them may not have learned the skills of communicating in a different way (e.g. signing or the use of communication boards).

Practice question

Do you, and/or others in your area of practice have the ability to communicate differently with those with speech, language or communication difficulties?

Because of their disability, this group of children and young people may be dependent on others (i.e. parents and carers) for support with activities of daily living, including intimate care. Furthermore, it is important to note that professionals and others working with families with a disabled child or young person can develop very intensive relationships with parents, and over-identify with them, with the result that it becomes difficult both to acknowledge, and to respond to, concerns about the child's safety and well-being. Although this chapter concerns the sexual abuse of children and young people, it is timely to reinforce the message that children and young people with disabilities are more likely to suffer from *all* forms of maltreatment: physical abuse, emotional abuse, sexual abuse and neglect. However, in relation to sexual abuse, Murray and Osborne (2009) make some noteworthy points in relation to the blocks that can prevent professionals from being open to the possibility of this form of abuse. These include the denial of the child or young person's sexuality and/or confusing behaviours that may be indicative of sexual abuse with those associated with the disability.

 Child's perspective

Jodie needs to be safe and to feel safe. Her experience of sexual abuse made her feel confused and 'dirty' and her condition means that she is finding it difficult to communicate with her mother or other family members about what happened, or to make sense of it. Her mother and father are cross, upset and anxious and although her thought processes are somewhat muddled, she associates their emotional state with her own wrongdoing.

The child protection plan

As we noted in Chapter 4, the decision at an ICPC to make a child or young person subject to a formal child protection plan is determined by the questions of whether they have suffered significant harm, and whether or not they are likely to be at risk of suffering significant harm in the future. The local authority takes responsibility for holding and updating a list of children and young people who are subject to a child protection plan, and there is a new system in place in England to ensure links between these data and clinical information systems in NHS urgent care settings and services (CP-IS). This system also enables the sharing of information in relation to names of looked-after children and pregnant women who have a pre-birth child protection plan. Professionals who need to ascertain the child protection status of a child or young person can also contact their local authority children's social care department (including the emergency duty service that operates outside of office hours) for this information.

The primary purposes of a child protection plan are to:

* ensure the child is safe from harm and prevent him or her from suffering further harm;
* promote the child's health and development; and
* support the family and wider family members to safeguard and promote the welfare of their child, provided it is in the best interests of the child.

(HM Government 2015a:45)

The child protection plan outlines an overall aim, as well as a number of short- and long-term actions and objectives for professionals and the family, aimed at reducing the likelihood of further harm. Arrangements are put in place to monitor the safety and well-being of the child (or children) and the compliance with the plan. A child protection plan is a formal document in which the following are agreed and recorded:

* actions to be undertaken/services to be provided;
* frequency/length of service;
* person/agency responsible;
* date of commencement;
* planned outcomes/progress to be achieved by next review.

There should be a clear contingency for failures to deliver or achieve actions and objectives and to escalate concerns, if necessary. By signing up to the child protection plan, families are providing a written agreement to work together with professionals to safeguard and promote the welfare of their child.

Child protection plans are monitored (and, if necessary, refined) by a 'core group' comprising the allocated social worker, the child or young person (if appropriate), the parents or carers (and possibly other family members) and key professionals involved with the child and family. The responsibility for chairing the core group and managing the plan normally sits with the local authority children's social care department, although in some areas this role is undertaken by the NSPCC. Accountability for delivering the plan rests with all the members of the core group, including the family.

The child and family should be fully informed as to the reasons and purpose of the child protection plan and advice will be provided about access to advocacy and support services. Meetings of the core group normally take place on a 6-weekly basis, between the dates of the ICPC and the RCPCs (see Chapter 7). The core group will have a contingency plan to be followed if family circumstances change and there is a greater threat to the child's safety.

Jodie's child protection plan

In Jodie's (and her siblings') case, the core group comprises Marcus, as the health professional who has the most frequent contact with the family, along with:

*   Jodie's parents and an aunt;
*   the lead social worker (who will be the 'key worker');
*   a social worker from the children with disabilities team;
*   the designated officer for safeguarding children (DOSC) from Jodie's special school;
*   a school nurse;
*   a health visitor and an early years worker.

A child protection plan will be drawn up for each of the children. The plan for Jodie, below, includes an outline of her health and developmental needs.

Action	Person/agency responsible	Outcomes
There will be 2-weekly planned joint visits to monitor Jodie's well-being	Key worker, children's social care and learning disability nurse, health provider	Jodie's welfare will be safeguarded and promoted

Action	Person/agency responsible	Outcomes
There will be alternate-week unannounced visits to assess Jodie's well-being and her parents' compliance with the requirements of the plan	Key worker, children's social care	Parents will comply with the child protection plan Jodie's welfare will be safeguarded and promoted
Jodie will receive an enhanced package of care that includes the delivery of a 'safe-touch' programme by [date]	School nurse, health provider and DOSC, special school	Jodie will have an awareness of her right to physical integrity and an enhanced ability to protect herself
Damian's contact with Jodie will be supervised at all times	Parents and aunt to Jodie, mother to Damian	Jodie will be protected from further risk of sexual abuse
The frequency of provision of respite care to be reviewed	Key worker, social worker, disability team and parents	Respite care provided is proportionate to Jodie's needs and the needs of the family at a time of additional stress
Staff at the hospice are aware of the child protection plan	Key worker and hospice staff	Staff are enabled to be vigilant regarding any additional concerns about Jodie's safety and well-being

The over-arching aim of the child protection plan is to ensure that Jodie and her siblings do not suffer future harm and a range of measures are put in place, including asking the family not to allow Damian to have unsupervised access to the children. Key to the core group, Marcus is able to provide advice on Jodie's condition, her health and developmental needs and assist other professionals in communicating with her. This includes supporting professionals who are helping Jodie in understanding 'safe touch'. Marcus is supported in his safeguarding role by his manager and clinical supervisor. The plan will be monitored and reviewed by the core group and progress reported to the RCPC.

Practice point

Marcus should seek regular child protection supervision to ensure that he is able to remain focused on the need to safeguard and promote the welfare of Jodie and her siblings. Given the complexity of the family situation,

and a genuine feeling of compassion for Natasha and Simon, it is important that the children's needs and interests are placed at the centre of
professionals' assessments and interventions.

Case 2 continued

In becoming involved in Jodie's case, Marcus finds himself questioning the
safeguarding and child protection knowledge and understanding of the children's hospice staff, some of whom have found it difficult to acknowledge the
abuse that has taken place. He is also concerned to find that the organization's
internal safeguarding children policy and procedures document appears to
be quite superficial. While the document provides guidance on what to do if
there are concerns that a child is being maltreated, as well as details of how
to seek further advice and make a referral to the local children's social care
department, it is disappointingly 'thin' on the particular risks of maltreatment
faced by children and young people with disabilities. Marcus believes that this
is an important omission because these children are a group who make up an
increasingly large proportion of the children and families in their care. At the
current time, the clinical lead takes a 'named' responsibility as part of their
portfolio of duties, but has limited time to undertake the professional development and multi-agency networking required for this role.

Marcus' experiences of the child protection processes surrounding Jodie
and her family have made him reflect on the readiness and ability of the LSCB's
partners to recognize and respond to concerns that a child with a disability
is being harmed. Marcus is also aware that for many families with disabled
young people facing transition to adult services, including residential care,
there is a need to ensure that safeguarding adult policies and procedures are
also in place locally. Drawing on the evidence base for practice and policy outlined by Murray and Osborne (2009), and with the support of his manager, the
LSCB chair and the designated nurse from the local CCG, Marcus proposes the
following objectives at his annual appraisal and review:

- to become the named nurse for the children's hospice;
- to revise and update the organization's internal safeguarding children
  policy and procedures;
- to undertake to develop a programme of in-house safeguarding children
  training and to ensure that staff requiring level-three training (RCPCH 2014)
  are able to access the inter-agency safeguarding training provided by the LSCB;
- to support the LSCB chair in working with a 'task and finish' group to
  develop an inter-agency protocol to support good practice for safeguarding disabled children and young people across local partners;

- to join the LSCB standing committee responsible for monitoring, scrutiny and evaluation of practice to ensure that the particular needs of disabled children are met;
- to establish a link with the Local Adult Safeguarding Board to support safety of disabled young people at the point of transition into adult services.

Markers of good practice: the role of the learning disability nurse

Marcus' role in safeguarding Jodie and her family is both to provide ongoing care and support, and also to act as an advocate and expert. His skills and knowledge are vital to ensure that the child protection plan achieves its aims, objectives and actions to safeguard and promote the welfare of all the children in the family.

He is a member of the core group and will ensure that he prioritizes attendance and produces reports, which he shares with the family prior to any meetings. He will also attend the RCPC.

Marcus also recognizes the potential for improvements to safeguarding children, young people and adults with disabilities and takes action to influence and transform practice. In doing so, he is practising within his professional remit to work cooperatively to preserve the safety of those receiving care (NMC 2015).

Case 3: Stewart – an adult client who discloses activity that is linked with child sexual abuse

Stewart is a 38-year-old divorced father of two, who suffers from recurrent manic depression. He is cared for by a community mental health team led by Georgiou, a registered nurse (mental health). Stewart is currently unemployed, has major debt issues and has recently admitted to 'drinking [alcohol] to excess'. This is having a big impact on his treatment and his present state of mental and physical health. Georgiou, who has taken on the role of mental health care coordinator, undertakes a home visit to make an assessment. Stewart presents as pale, tearful and anxious, and explains that his estranged ex-wife has sought to further reduce his contact with his children. During the visit Stewart admits that he is accessing the internet on a regular basis to watch child pornography – for which he has to pay – and that he is also passing on images of young boys to others who indulge in this activity. Stewart begs Georgiou not to record or share this information with anyone else, adding that it has been shared by him in strict confidence.

Practice question

Should Georgiou respect his client's right to confidentiality?

Viewing online images of children

Involving children in the production of, or watching of, sexual images is within the statutory definition of child sexual abuse (HM Government 2015a). According to a report from the Child Exploitation and Online Protection centre (CEOP), the viewing of indecent images of children is 'alarmingly common-place', with compelling evidence that those who view such images are a risk to children (CEOP 2012). The images themselves represent the multiple and significant harm suffered by the children who are clearly subject to abuse at the time of creating the image, and their re-victimization with each viewing. According to the CEOP, investigations into those who view online images have led to the discovery of victims who have suffered years of offline sexual abuse. These victims include offenders' own children, other family members or the children's friends. The profile of the largest group of perpetrators features unemployed white males, with the second most common group being those who are employed in schools or care work. The CEOP recognizes the vital role of statutory agencies in supporting the police in the detection of offending.

Many parents and carers express concerns about children and young people's use of the internet via their computers or mobile devices. It is clear that we are now in an age where children and young people have almost constant access to social media. In addition to their role in tackling online abuse, the CEOP sponsors a website ('ThinkUKnow')[2] that offers tailored guidance for professionals, parents and children themselves on protection from child sexual abuse and exploitation (both on- and offline) and cyber-bullying. The CEOP site also has a facility to access help and advice and to make reports about online activity that may indicate crimes against children and young people.

Case 3 continued

Georgiou contacts his line manager for advice and support in reporting the matter to the police. Given the fact that his concerns would meet the threshold for 'public interest', details of Stewart's disclosure of accessing child pornography are passed to the local police child abuse referral unit.

Although Stewart has requested his right to confidentiality in this matter, Georgiou has taken the correct decision in reporting the disclosure to the police. This apparent breach of confidentiality meets the NMC code (2015) requirement that information is shared because it is believed that someone is at risk of harm. The sharing of information without consent would also be supported

[2]https://www.thinkuknow.co.uk/.

by information-sharing guidance as being in the public interest. In this case, information is shared with the police promptly, as it relates to criminal activity (HM Government 2015b). In their enquiries, the police will have to consider Stewart's access to children, including his own. There may be a need for them to work with children's social care services to initiate a Section 47 investigation as it is possible that Stewart's children (and their friends and other children in the wider family) have been party to watching the child sexual abuse or even been caught up in the production of images. Stewart is currently not in work, but if his employment or any volunteering activities involved working with children and young people (e.g. Scout leader), then this would have to be addressed in conjunction with the local authority designated officer (LADO) whose role it is to investigate allegations made concerning people who work or volunteer with children and young people (HM Government 2015a).

Markers of good practice: the role of the mental health nurse

Before the establishment of any therapeutic relationship, it is advisable to set out with the client the professional boundaries, duties and responsibilities in relation to confidentiality. Georgiou recognizes that he has to share information with the police following the disclosure. He seeks support from his line manager, but equally could have approached his organization's safeguarding children leads.

Georgiou completes clear, contemporaneous records of the events and his actions, with particular regard to the admission of criminal activity that was causing harm to others and his decision to share information with the police (NMC 2015).

Summary

This chapter has considered child sexual abuse. As noted in the statutory definition, sexual abuse may involve physical contact or non-contact activities such as involving the child in looking at sexual images or grooming in preparation for abuse. An important message is that children may not be aware at the time that what is happening to them is abusive. Three scenarios have been presented. The first scenario concerned Maryam who was experiencing peer-related abuse that included ongoing threats of posting images of her on social media. The second scenario concerned Jodie, who has a progressive and life-limiting condition and a range of disabilities that have made her vulnerable to sexual abuse. The third scenario demonstrated the need to take action in informing the police following a disclosure by an adult mental health services client that they were accessing child pornography online. The nursing staff involved in these fictitious scenarios were a sexual health nurse, a learning disabilities nurse and an adult mental health nurse. A range of safeguarding actions were described. The scenarios demonstrate the importance of information-sharing, as well as the very positive actions that nurses and midwives can take in ensuring the safety and well-being of individual clients or patients, their families and communities.

Key points

- Children and young people who are sexually abused experience difficulty in telling their story. Victims are not always aware that what is happening to them is abusive.
- The effects of child sexual abuse are enduring and may be lifelong.
- Children who are disabled have a threefold risk of being abused, but are under-represented in safeguarding systems.
- Confidentiality in a patient-client relationship is *not* absolute; this should be explained to clients at the outset of any therapeutic relationship.
- In the case of Stewart, the 'public interest' would be served by reporting his online activity to the police.

6

Child sexual exploitation

Learning outcomes

This chapter will help you to:

- Understand the features of child sexual exploitation (CSE) as a form of child maltreatment, including the risk factors.
- Develop your understanding of the particular challenges of identification of this form of abuse.
- Identify the links between CSE and risk-taking behaviours, including the misuse of alcohol and drugs.
- Ensure that children and young people who are victims of CSE are seen as children first and foremost.
- Understand how to escalate concerns to ensure the safety and protection of a child or young person.

Introduction

The issue of CSE has been prominent at the time of writing the second edition of this 'practical guide' and therefore it may be of no surprise to readers that a decision was made to include a stand-alone chapter on this type of child maltreatment. This is a form of maltreatment that is both pernicious in its effects and that also raises some fundamental questions about the way in which children and young people (especially 'bad' children and young people) are viewed by those providing their care. Above all, the experiences of children who have been victims of CSE should help to embed the principles outlined earlier in this book – i.e. the importance of listening to the voice the child, believing what they say and seeking to understand their daily lived experiences. The chapter begins by providing an overview of CSE as a form of child sexual abuse, and highlights some of the current policies and work-streams that are aiming to seek better understanding in tackling the issues, as well as the evidence of significant harm that CSE has on the victims. We then reflect on some of the learning from the serious case reviews and enquiries that have been undertaken, and how the themes that have arisen from this work can influence practice improvements. The opportunities that nurses and midwives have to recognize and respond to CSE are self-evident, but it is not, as the evidence suggests, always as straightforward in practice as it seems in the literature.

Three case scenarios are presented:

- Case 1: Lacey, aged 16 years, has been brought to the emergency department (ED) having taken a cocktail of prescribed medication and alcohol. She is difficult to rouse. This is the fourth time that she has presented as a result of self-harming behaviour. Lacey refuses to provide details of the two older men who are hovering in the waiting room and asking when she will be 'let out'.
- Case 2: Zara, who is 14 years of age, is seeking her second termination of pregnancy. She tells the staff at the young persons' contraception and sexual health service that she got drunk at a party.
- Case 3: Elsa, who is 15 years old, has been in and out of care. She is now placed in a secure children's home in an attempt to prevent yet another episode of going missing. A nurse from the looked-after children team is due to meet Elsa for a routine health review.

Child sexual exploitation as a form of child sexual abuse

CSE is a form of child sexual abuse that is explicitly recognized in the UNCRC 1989 (see Chapter 1). It is a global issue and one that the UK has sought to robustly address through the provision of supplementary safeguarding and child protection guidance (HM Government 2009; DfE 2012), and the recent commissioning of a number of enquiry reports and evidence appraisals (e.g. Berelowitz et al. 2013; HM Government 2013; House of Commons Home Affairs Committee 2013; Pearce 2013; DH/Health Working Group 2014). Furthermore, current statutory guidance now reflects the groundswell of public and ministerial pressure to tackle this form of maltreatment, presumably fuelled by the publicity that has followed the publication of a number of high-profile serious case reviews and reports into localized grooming of victims and CSE perpetrated by gangs and groups, as well as the ongoing enquiries into celebrity sexual abuse 'scandals'. It is difficult to be certain as to the prevalence of this form of abuse, but once enquiries are made, victims may be identified, with many more at risk (Berelowitz et al. 2013). As a result of the increased interest and profile of CSE, LSCBs are now required to undertake regular assessments and scrutiny of board partners' responses to CSE and to include evidence of this work in their annual reports (HM Government 2015a).

Practice point

In the past, the notion of sexual exploitation of children was, for the most part, referred to as 'child prostitution'. However, this label is completely inappropriate and fails to recognize that the child or young person is essentially a victim who is being abused by perpetrators who hold power and control over them. CSE is a largely gendered issue (i.e. girls are usually the victims and boys or men are usually the perpetrators) and; in contrast to public opinion, both victims and perpetrators reflect the rich heritage and diversity of the population.

CSE is an issue that needs to be framed within a children's rights framework and, in particular, seeks to balance the protective rights of children and young people with their right to freely experience their age-appropriate developmental needs into adulthood. However, there have to be checks and balances to ensure that they are fundamentally safe and well. In supplementary guidance to *Working Together* the following definition of CSE is given:

> Sexual exploitation of children and young people under 18 involves exploitative situations, contexts and relationships where young people (or a third person or persons) receive 'something' (e.g. food, accommodation, drugs, alcohol, cigarettes, affection, gifts, money) as a result of them performing, and/or another or others performing on them, sexual activities. Child sexual exploitation can occur through the use of technology without the child's immediate recognition; for example being persuaded to post sexual images on the Internet/mobile phones without immediate payment or gain. In all cases, those exploiting the child/young person have power over them by virtue of their age, gender, intellect, physical strength and/or economic or other resources. Violence, coercion and intimidation are common, involvement in exploitative relationships being characterized in the main by the child or young person's limited availability of choice resulting from their social/economic and/or emotional vulnerability.
>
> (HM Government 2009:9)

Although the risk of sexual exploitation applies to any child or young person, certain groups are reported to be at greater risk; these include those with a history of maltreatment or other adverse events in their childhood (such as living with parental mental health problems, substance misuse or domestic violence and abuse), children in care, those who truant from school or run away from home or placement, immigrants and those with learning difficulties or disabilities. The risk may also apply to their friends. There are also links with forced marriage, in itself an issue that affects mainly younger victims.[1] Boys as well as girls are targeted and for some victims the coerced sexual activity can lead to confusion of sexual orientation (HM Government 2009). In contrast with a commonly held view of prostitutes offering their wares on street corners, children and young people who are subject to sexual exploitation are usually

---

[1] https://www.gov.uk/forced-marriage provides help for victims and resources for professionals on this matter.

hidden from view in premises that have been secured for this purpose. Where CSE has been identified, the role of fast food and taxi/mini-cab businesses has been mentioned, but this is not the only scenario. It is shocking to find that those organizing the abuse may include family members, as well as other adults. Young people themselves can also be perpetrators of CSE and a finding from some of the reviews of cases is that perpetrators will put pressure on their victims to recruit their friends into becoming future victims of CSE. The age range of victims has been reported to be from 11 years to young women entering adulthood. The perpetrators are generally older, but as noted above, some will be below the age of 18. Perpetrators can act alone or in gangs or groups.

The response to the sexual exploitation of children adds additional challenges to LSCB partners, including health services, in that this form of abuse crosses geographical boundaries, as well as UK borders. Some of the victims have been found to have been trafficked for the purposes of sexual exploitation (see also HM Government 2008b). The ever-expanding use of technology and mobile devices adds another important dimension to grooming via the internet and social media. Health professionals working with children, young people and their families can help to contribute to preventative activities through ensuring their own knowledge of techology is robust and providing signposting to sources of advice and support to those concerned about their children's e-safety.

The outcomes for children and young people who have been sexually exploited can be extremely poor and have been linked to long-term physical, psychological and sexual harm (HM Government 2009). For some individuals, it can lead to the loss of their life, either through being murdered (Jay 2014) or by committing suicide. Serious and enduring consequences have been reported to include the following:

- unwanted pregnancy;
- sexually transmitted infections, including transmission of the human immunodeficiency virus (HIV);
- gynaecological problems;
- relationship difficulties (family and intimate partner);
- feeling of worthlessness leading to self-harm and eating disorders;
- substance misuse and addiction;
- entering a life of prostitution as an adult.

It is therefore paramount that any concerns that a child or young person may be being sexually exploited are shared and actions taken to safeguard them from further harm. Addressing CSE is clearly a public health imperative.

The role of nurses and midwives

Nurses and midwives are recognized to have a role in the prevention of CSE through the promotion of 'safe and healthy' choices, as well as the identification and referral of victims and perpetrators. In some areas, specialist multi-disciplinary CSE teams are being set up and will include specialist nurses in their make-up. There is clearly a need to develop health professionals' knowledge, skills and competence in this form of abuse. The report by Berelowitz *et al.* (2013) outlines several recommendations that directly reflect the training requirements of health professionals. These include the need to understand the nature of CSE, to be able to spot the warning signs, to be able to refer to services for CSE and to have access to supervision and support in practice. While acknowledging that they are not in a position of recommending the details of any particular training package, the authors of the report suggest that this should highlight CSE in general as well as CSE in gangs and groups, and that any training should be delivered in the broader context of safeguarding, child sexual abuse and gender-based violence. The issue of inclusion of CSE on pre-registration curricula is a point made by the DH Working Group (2014). Similarly to the current guidance (HM Government 2009), Berelowitz *et al.*'s report also notes the breadth of health services that may come into contact with children who are victims of CSE, including emergency and urgent care departments, CAMHS, contraception and sexual health services, drug and alcohol services, general practice, midwifery and health visiting (and presumably the Family Nurse Partnership, FNP) and sexual assault and referral centres (SARCs). An understanding of the risk factors and indicators of CSE is vital in informing assessment. The use of the Sexual Exploitation Risk Assessment Framework (SERAF) first developed by Barnardo's in Wales is gaining momentum across many LSCB areas (Barnardo's Cymru 2013). The SERAF provides a structured format that can be used to gather and organize information and make an informed decision on the level of risk a young person is facing, to share the assessment and help to ensure a timely and helpful response.

Practice point

Sexual exploitation of children and young people is a criminal activity. Information-sharing is vital. Nurses and midwives are protected in sharing information if they have concerns about harm to an individual, even in the absence of consent to share. The sharing of timely and proportionate information is supported by the government guidance highlighted in Chapter 1 (HM Government 2015b) and also by the professional code (NMC 2015).

Learning from case reviews

The NSPCC provide a useful summary of the learning from serious case reviews that have been commissioned by LSCBs following cases of CSE (NSPCC 2013). An important message from this briefing is that CSE can be hard to recognize and respond to because young people (at least at the outset) do not themselves recognize the abuse and believe themselves to be in loving relationships. Added to this is the recognition that disclosure is unlikely for a number of reasons. These may include fear of, or loyalty to, the perpetrator and a lack of trust in, or fear of, those in authority. Those who do seek help are not always responded to appropriately.

The reviews highlight the importance of practitioners being able to recognize risk factors for CSE (see above). The NSPCC suggest that practitioners should be aware of the 'warning signs' of CSE, including under-age sexual activity, sexual health concerns, teenage pregnancy, involvement in crime, concerning relationships (especially with unknown adults), alcohol and drug use, missing from home and truancy and exclusion and disengagement from school. Many victims were viewed as being troublemakers and responses include criminalizing their behaviour, rather than ensuring protection and support.

Most crucially, the NSPCC argue that professionals providing contraception and sexual health services should consider whether there are child protection issues, including possible sexual exploitation, *whenever* they become aware of underage sexual activity. Assessments, they add, should include the wider picture and professional judgement on capacity to consent and should take into account the possibility of grooming and coercion. Importantly, they note that in some cases, CSE involving 16- and 17-year-olds was not recognized simply because the young people were presumed to be in consensual relationships.

Three high-profile cases are worthy of additional mention here: Rochdale, Rotherham and Oxford. The events in these three places have been subject to much exposure in the media. However, a note of caution here – CSE is not limited to towns and cities in any particular geographical locality, it is likely to occur everywhere (Berelowitz *et al.* 2013).

The Rochdale case involved the CSE of a large number of victims over a period of several years. Perpetrators were linked to take-away premises and taxi firms. The review of the case referenced the experiences of 'Suzie' (Rochdale Borough Safeguarding Children Board 2012). Suzie, who used alcohol and drugs, became pregnant as a result of her abuse. After the baby was born, the attention of agencies turned from Suzie (who was still a child) to child protection concerns about the baby in the context of male visitors to the home. This meant that she felt under pressure from professionals regarding her parenting skills. During the time period subject to the review, lead statutory agencies were under pressure from increased referrals, which were thought to have resulted from the publicity surrounding the Peter Connelly (Baby P.) case. Their attention was subsequently focused on the needs of younger children, with CSE not necessarily viewed as a 'mainstream child protection issue'. According to the review, the victims of CSE were seen to be making their own choices and engaging in consensual sexual activity. Victims' evidence is included in an addendum to the report; an important message from this evidence was that when victims did seek help from children's social care and/or the police they reported that nothing changed for them.

The enquiry into CSE in Rotherham was led by Alexis Jay and published in 2014. The report suggests that as many as 1400 children were victims of CSE between 1997 and 2013; graphic details are provided of the rape and torture of many of the victims, especially at the point at which they may have decided to disclose what is happening to them to the authorities. While the report is mainly centred on the responses of the local politicians, police and children's social care to CSE, some commentary is given about the role of health services. This includes a positive reflection on the appointment of a specialist nurse to the CSE team and the establishment of CSE care pathways for children and young people attending contraception and sexual health services. The report made a recommendation to health services to improve the provision of longer term counselling and support for victims (Jay 2014).

The serious case review into CSE in Oxfordshire was published in 2015. The report author, Alan Bedford, noted that the events were allowed to happen (as elsewhere in the country) in part because of a lack of knowledge and processes in place at the time, but also because in many cases there had been a lack of 'curiosity' and even 'common sense'. As in other reviews, he found plentiful evidence of victim-blaming, as well as services that viewed the young people as either competent adults or as children who were essentially engaged in bad behaviour. The description of the rape and torture of the children is extremely distressing, and the degree of depravity extreme. Many of the victims were heavily drugged and the multiple abuse by gangs of men sometimes lasted for several days. While symptoms of their CSE were generally treated and responded to adequately by health professionals, Bedford found that there was a lack of enquiry into how these symptoms came about. In summarizing his assessment, he commented on the existence of 'a professional mindset which could not grasp that the victims' ability to say no had been totally eroded' (Oxfordshire Safeguarding Children Board 2015:2). A particular message for nurses and midwives is that there is a need to join up information from a range of provision, because the victims accessed health services (including those that offered terminations of pregnancy) from different health care providers, which prevented any pattern of attendances or presentations to be determined. In finding that victims had accessed alcohol and drugs services, the author also neatly described the use of alcohol for CSE victims as initially a gift; then to weaken resistance; and finally to anaesthetize following their trauma.

Case 1: Lacey – fourth time in the emergency department

Lacey, who is nearly 17 years of age, has been brought to the ED in a semi-comatose condition. This is the fourth time in the past year that she has presented. It transpires that she has been drinking heavily for 'two or three days' and 'taken some pills'. Lacey is admitted to the observation bay for treatment with IV fluids and monitoring. Bloods are taken for toxicology. Staff have noticed that Lacey's appearance and presentation is somewhat poor; she is unwashed and her copious make-up is smudged. It is difficult not to notice that her body odour is strong and unpleasant. Blood and vomit are ingrained on her clothing. When roused, Lacey refuses to give a clear history and tells staff that she was brought in by 'a couple of friends' she was partying with. She does not want her mother informed of her admission, and anyway she has lost her mobile, and cannot remember her mother's number off by heart. She tells staff that she is OK and that her friends will take her home.

 Child's perspective

Lacey is a victim of CSE. She has been put under some pressure from her abusers to 'keep quiet', which she is content to do, providing that they continue to look after her and stop threatening her with another beating. She has mainly enjoyed the partying and it feels good to have been seen to be attractive to her boyfriend and his friends. She just wishes that he would keep her all to himself. She thinks the ED staff are extremely nosy.

Developing a chronology

Sandra, the triage nurse, was on duty when Lacey was admitted the first time. She remembers her because at that time she came in with quite marked bruising to her face. Sandra calls up the records from Lacey's previous attendances and makes a note of the dates and the presentations. Although one of the records is quite scanty, she surmises that each of the presentations has an element of concern and moreover there does not seem to be a record of any parental details in any of the next of kin boxes. Sandra bleeps the Trust's named nurse for safeguarding children.

Case 1 continued

Meanwhile, the two men who accompanied Lacey keep asking when they can go in to see her. They look anxious and distracted and refuse to give their names, telling the receptionist that it is 'none of her f***ing business'. Luckily, the department is relatively quiet and Sandra asks the team caring for Lacey if they can possibly hold onto her until she and the safeguarding lead have had a discussion and an opportunity to undertake some further enquiries. This will include trying to contact a parent or carer. Lacey's presentation is not one of a 'competent young person' and although she is over the age of 16 years, she is still legally a child.

Lacey's mother is eventually contacted and somewhat reluctantly agrees to come in after she has found someone to look after her three younger children (half-siblings to Lacey). She is informed about the referral to children's social care and the reasons for this. By this time the men accompanying Lacey to the ED have left the building. The relationship between Lacey and her mother appears to be strained; her mother confides that she has been getting increasingly cross about Lacey's frequent episodes of 'going missing'. It also transpires that Lacey is known to the police because of 'petty crime' (shoplifting in the local chemist shop). A good response to the referral to statutory agencies will be one that is responsive to the cluster of indicators that point to Lacey's risk from sexual exploitation and perhaps help to rescue her, and other children, from their abuse.

Markers of good practice: the role of the triage nurse

Sandra has recognized that Lacey is a child who may be in need of help. She has taken time to contextualize the latest admission to the ED both in terms of the pattern of attendances and also the other reasons for attending.

Sandra seeks supervision with the named nurse and a decision is made that a referral will be made to children's social care. Lacey's permission for the referral will be sought, but if it is refused then staff will explain why it is necessary to contact them as people are concerned for her safety and welfare.

It will be important to ensure that the information that is shared is proportionate, but clearly outlines the reasons why there is concern that Lacey may be a victim of CSE. Sandra also seeks out the two men who accompanied Lacey to the ED, to ask if they can provide details of their relationship with her. However, they appear to have left the department.

Sandra completes a written referral to children's social care to follow a telephone referral. A copy is placed in Lacey's ED records and her main case notes.

The school nursing service is contacted, but at the current time they are not commissioned to provide a service to post-compulsory education providers.

Case 2: Zara attends a young person's contraception and sexual health clinic

Zara, who is 14 years of age, is seeking her second termination of pregnancy. She has attended the clinic with a nervous-looking female teacher but appears nonchalant and calm. She looks older than her 14 years. Zara tells the staff at the clinic that she got drunk at a party and is not sure of the name of the 'lad' she had sex with.

Ana, a specialist young person's contraception and sexual health (CASH) nurse has recently moved from an adjoining Trust. This is a new service and she is keen to ensure that the young people who attend are made to feel welcome and respected (DH 2011). However, she has read up on safeguarding and child protection in preparation for her interview, and is determined to ensure that no child in need of safeguarding 'slips through the net'. The clinic manager and receptionist have been in post for many years; they tell Ana they 'have seen it all before'. She is finding them rather intimidating. They are also clear that they pride themselves in offering young people a 'totally confidential service' – after all, they add, 'we are known to be trusted by the youngsters in this area.'

Practice question

What is your view of Ana's approach and that of the more experienced manager and receptionist?

Ana is concerned about the level of awareness of safeguarding and child protection in the clinic, and in the wider CASH service in the area. She is also conscious that many of the clinics are in remote places. Some are run as 'pop ups' (also known as 'clinic in a box'). Nearly all the medical and nursing staff are working part-time, combining work with other job roles and/or responsibilities such as caring for a young family or looking after elderly parents. Ana has just booked onto the Trust's induction training and decides that she will find an opportunity at the coffee break to discuss concerns about safeguarding children awareness with the named nurse who will be delivering the introductory session on safeguarding at this training. Meanwhile, her concerns about practice are mounting, especially when she sees the records that were completed at the time of Zara's previous attendance.

Whistle-blowing and safeguarding practice

Although she has only just arrived, Ana has recognized that there may well be a culture of poor safeguarding and child protection practice within the CASH service. While she accepts that staff may be motivated by pride in delivering a 'confidential service', she is concerned that this may not be in the best interests of the young people who access the service. Her decision to challenge the status quo is not a comfortable one, especially given her recent arrival in the Trust, and her relative lack of experience when compared with her colleagues. However, it does fit with the expectation of the statutory guidance that health services will have whistle-blowing procedures in place that enable issues about safeguarding and promoting the welfare of children to be addressed (HM Government 2015a).

A decision is made to conduct a retrospective audit of the case notes of all the children and young people attending the CASH service in the previous

6 months. The standards for the audit will be based on the LSCB CSE protocol and incorporate elements of the SERAF tool. The named nurse, who is also recently in post, will support the audit. The named nurse, in turn, will share her concerns with the designated nurse at supervision. It is likely that commissioners will seek to use their powers within contracting and quality surveillance to monitor the situation and to drive up standards in the service. This will include checking that CASH staff have updated their safeguarding and child protection training in line with recommended practice (RCPCH 2014).

Case 2 continued

Meanwhile, the immediate safeguarding needs of Zara have to be addressed. Ana will seek to undertake an assessment to help them both understand the risky behaviour that she is currently engaging in. A systematic approach, drawing on the assessment framework (HM Government 2015a:22), will help to identify wider unmet needs and inform a referral to children's social care. The use of a genogram ('family tree') will help to identify who has parental responsibility for Zara and enable a discussion about her family life. Her teacher is asked to wait.

 Child's perspective

Zara may be a victim of CSE. Although she is calm, she is, in reality, extremely frightened about the reaction of her mother and stepfather to this pregnancy. Her previous termination was as a result of a rape by a family friend, when she was just 12 years of age. At the time her family blamed her for 'leading him on'. This pregnancy has arisen because of a new friendship with a 19-year-old, who she knows her mother would not approve of, but he is kind and generous and she is determined to keep meeting him in secret. Zara finds Ana easy to talk to.

Markers of good practice: the role of the young person's sexual health nurse

Ana has ensured that she has a good understanding of her safeguarding and child protection responsibilities and knows how to seek advice and support.

Ana recognizes that the practice within the CASH service is placing children and young people at risk. She is prepared to address these concerns in a timely manner. This meets with requirements of the Trust's whistle-blowing policy and her responsibilities as a nurse (NMC 2015).

She also understands the role of audit in seeking to embed practice improvements.

Case 3: Elsa, who keeps going missing

Elsa, who is 15 years old, has been in and out of care because of a history of intra-familial physical abuse and neglect. She has not settled at her recent placement with new foster carers (whom she describes as bossy and fussy) and is now in a secure children's home in an attempt to prevent yet another episode of going missing. Juliet, a specialist nurse from the looked-after children team, who is allocated to the home, is due to meet Elsa for a routine health review in line with statutory requirements for looked-after children (RCN/RCPCH 2015). After meeting up on a day and at a time negotiated with Elsa, Juliet introduces herself. Elsa is more than aware of the need for these 'check-ups' and is keen to see if Juliet has brought along any spare condoms. The first thing that strikes Juliet is the fact that Elsa appears to be somewhat under-weight, and her skin is in poor condition. She also appears to be distracted and keeps looking at her phone. Juliet, who is popular with staff at the home, has been told that they have recently noticed that cars from a local mini-cab firm have been driving up and down the street and slowing down when they pass the building.

Practice question

If you were undertaking this health review, what would be your key concerns about Elsa's health and well-being?

There are some worrying indicators about Elsa's well-being and safety. These include: the frequency at which she is going missing; her weight loss and poor physical health (possibly indicating substance misuse); the fact that she is engaging in underage sexual activity; her preoccupation with looking at her phone (albeit that this is common in this age group); and the context of concerns raised by staff in relation to the taxi drivers (which may be entirely coincidental). However, there are indicators of concern and Juliet will try to gather as much information as she can, explain her concerns to Elsa and seek safeguarding and child protection supervision from her colleague in the safeguarding children team. She asks the staff if they have reported the cruising taxi-cabs to the police.

Child's perspective

Elsa is being subject to CSE by a local organized gang. This has been going on for some months. She is now being given amphetamines, to which she is becoming addicted. What started as her first 'proper boyfriend' has turned into an abusive and threatening situation; she is very frightened and has had no trusted adult to share her story with. No one will believe this, but she once found herself in a strange town and did not know how she got there. She had to beg for her train fare home.

Markers of good practice: the role of the looked-after children's nurse

Keen to establish a good relationship from the start, Juliet offered a time and place to meet with Elsa and undertake her health review.

Juliet has established good working relationships with staff in the home. However, this does not include sharing any clinical information without the consent of the young people in her care.

Juliet's health reviews are holistic – seeking to assess physical, psychological, behavioural and emotional dimensions of young people's well-being (RCN/RCPCH 2015).

She understands that as a result of becoming 'looked-after' parental responsibility is shared between Elsa's birth mother and the local authority. However, when she contacts Elsa's social worker, her concerns about CSE are minimized. With the support of the named nurse, and in accordance with LSCB procedures, Juliet escalates her concerns to a senior social work manager.

Summary

This chapter has provided an overview of CSE as a form of child sexual abuse, currently under the spotlight in the UK (and indeed globally). Nationally, a number of high-level workstreams have sought to better understand the risks for CSE and to develop strategies to prevent this exceedingly harmful form of child maltreatment. Locally, LSCBs have to formally report on actions they are taking to address CSE. Learning from national serious case reviews and enquiries has informed practitioner understanding, but any response needs to involve collaborative approaches across agencies and the engagement of children, young people and their families and communities.

Three scenarios have been presented. The first concerned Lacey, a 16-year-old who presented to the ED for the fourth time. In the context of concerns about her history and presentation, and the behaviours of two accompanying but unknown males, Sandra is concerned that Lacey may be a victim of CSE. The second case involves Zara, a 14 year old who presents for her second termination. Ana, a newly appointed CASH nurse, finds that safeguarding and child protection practice in the service is poor, and is concerned that it is placing children and young people at risk. She seeks to whistle-blow on what has been an entrenched culture over a long period of time. Finally, we met Elsa, a looked-after child who has been groomed by a gang of perpetrators of CSE. Juliet, the looked-after children's nurse, recognizes the possibility of CSE and, working with safeguarding leads, escalates her concerns about Elsa to managers in children's social care.

Key points

- CSE is pernicious in its effects and raises some fundamental questions about the way in which children and young people (especially 'bad' children and young people) are viewed.
- Those individuals presenting with symptoms of CSE need to have the cause of their symptoms identified.
- Children and young people are groomed into CSE; at least initially many of them will genuinely believe that they are in a loving and consensual relationship.
- Children and young people are victims of CSE, not 'child prostitutes'. Perpetrators are committing criminal acts.
- Nurses, midwives and health visitors can escalate their concerns about poor practice through reference to organizational whistle-blowing policies.
- In cases of professional disagreement, LSCB escalation policies apply. Advice and support can be given by named nurses and their teams.

7

Neglect

Learning outcomes

This chapter will help you to:

- Understand the features of neglect as a form of child maltreatment.
- Identify indicators that may be associated with neglect.
- Appreciate the challenges to recognizing and responding to neglect in practice.
- Make a professional contribution to a child protection review conference (CPRC), including supporting a decision to remove children's names from being subject to a formal child protection plan.

Introduction

Nurses, midwives and health visitors working with children, young people and their families may encounter neglect in the course of their practice. As with emotional abuse, context, rather than a specific event, underpins recognition of this form of maltreatment, although it frequently co-exists with other forms of child maltreatment. Drawing on the statutory guidance we begin by defining what is meant by 'neglect' and outlining some of the key indicators of concern. Throughout the chapter links are made to the evidence base for practice, as well as to safeguarding and child protection policy and procedures. Once again, three case scenarios are presented. These illustrate examples of child neglect and the practice implications for nurses, midwives and health visitors. The cases are fictitious, but based on reality.

- Case 1: Jack, a newborn baby, is at risk of neglect because of his mother's lifestyle. Christina, a community midwife, is anxious about his future well-being.
- Case 2: 18-month-old twins Courtney and Kendra presented at 9 months with 'faltering growth' and other physical and developmental indicators of neglect. They have subsequently been subject to a child protection plan and the case is due to be reviewed. Amanda, the health visitor, will attend the CPRC.

- Case 3: Logan, aged 4 years, was admitted to a paediatric intensive care unit with respiratory depression after accidentally ingesting one of his father's suboxone tablets. Molly, a substance misuse practitioner, has been supporting an investigation into the case.

It is important for health care staff to understand the seriousness of neglect and to be vigilant. Neglect is a significant, and preventable, cause of health and developmental difficulties for children and it can lead to childhood fatality.

Neglect

Neglect is a form of child maltreatment that is multi-faceted. Some of the child protection literature makes reference to 'emotional neglect' as well as 'physical neglect', but these often co-exist and both are subsumed within the statutory guidance definition:

> Neglect is the persistent failure to meet a child's basic physical and/or psychological needs, likely to result in the serious impairment of the child's health or development. Neglect may occur during pregnancy as a result of maternal substance abuse. Once a child is born, neglect may involve a parent or carer failing to:

- provide adequate food, clothing and shelter (including exclusion from home or abandonment);
- protect a child from physical and emotional harm or danger;
- ensure adequate supervision (including the use of inadequate caregivers); or
- ensure access to appropriate medical care or treatment.

> It may also include neglect of, or unresponsiveness to, a child's basic emotional needs.
>
> (HM Government 2015a:93)

Agreeing what is, and what is not, child neglect can be challenging. I have previously drawn attention to the ostensibly controversial work by Golden *et al.* (2003), who took the view that the use of the term 'neglect' was somewhat mild (Powell 2007). The authors' concerns were that the use of the concept suggested a *non-deliberate* failure to meet the needs of children through stress, competing priorities, lack of education and socioeconomic deprivation. Indeed, they argue that most parents will be guilty of neglect at some point, adding that it might actually be beneficial for children and young people's development into adulthood to experience not having all their needs met fully at all times.

By noting that in comparison with other forms of abuse neglect does not 'fit' with statutory procedures (that are designed to deal with an incident rather than a context) Golden *et al.* (2003) questioned the usefulness of a child protection approach for neglect. 'Mothers [*sic*]', they add, who are struggling with the challenges of parenting and adverse social and financial circumstances, are often aware that the care they are providing is not as good as it should be, but are less aware of the impact of this care on the child. In a similar vein, Gardner (2008) describes the concerns that many professionals have that in raising questions of neglect within families they may be seen to be blaming parents who are not 'intentionally abusive'. However, it is important to keep focused on the daily experiences of children. A report into research undertaken with children and young people who had experienced neglect spoke of the need for professionals to recognize and respond to their situation, reporting that neglect made them feel depressed, unloved and invisible (Action for Children 2014).

Compared with other forms of child maltreatment, neglect is evidently difficult to define and address. This is because it is clearly open to broader influences, heavily reliant on professional judgement and prone to discrepant parental interpretation. As we will find, these difficulties have contributed to the evidence to suggest that the professional response is frequently too little, too late (Brandon *et al.* 2014a; Ofsted 2014).

Prevalence of neglect

Radford *et al.* (2011) drew on a range of measures to describe the prevalence of self-reported neglect in childhood, and suggested reported rates of between 5 per cent (for children under 11 years of age) and 16 per cent for 18–24-year-olds, with 9 per cent of respondents meeting the researchers definition of 'severe' neglect based on victims' perception of their childhood experiences. As we noted in Chapter 3, the numbers of children and young people who are subject to a child protection plan have been rising in recent years, in tandem with a steep rise in overall referrals to children's social care. Neglect currently represents the largest proportion of those with a plan, at around 41 per cent of the total (DfE 2014a). The reasons for this could be that there is a genuine increase in neglect, or that practitioners are getting better at recognizing and responding to situations in which children's health and development are neglected. However, neglect was noted to be a feature in 60 per cent of serious case reviews (Brandon *et al.* 2012), with deaths of children attributed to a lack of supervision, accidental ingestion of drugs, drowning, falls, electrocution and fires, or in some cases in the context of co-sleeping with parents who had consumed drugs or alcohol. Many children who are subject to a serious case review are not known to the lead statutory agencies (i.e. children's social care), making it vital that nurses, midwives and health visitors, together with other providers of services to children, young people and their families are able to ensure recognition and a timely response (Brandon *et al.* 2014a).

Child neglect is widely acknowledged to be associated with parental difficulties including substance misuse, domestic violence and abuse, physical and mental health problems and learning disability – factors that lead to the provision of a range of services and opportunities to identify children's unmet needs.

Practice question

How can adults with learning disabilities be supported to parent well? On what basis should 'good enough' parenting by such individuals be assessed?

While the majority of families in poverty do not neglect their children, and neglect (especially emotional neglect) may feature in better off families, poor living conditions and social isolation together with the stress caused by the multiple demands of parenting are contributory factors. At a time of austerity in the UK (and elsewhere) the impact on children is concerning. As Brandon *et al.* (2014a) note, the current economic climate is undoubtedly challenging for both families and professionals and expenditure on services for children and families has not kept pace with the increasing demand for services.

Practice point

Disabled children, and those with a chronic illness, are known to be at particular risk of neglect. This may be due to family circumstance, service provision or society's attitudes to disability.

Impact of neglect

Neglect can impact on the health and development of children and young people at a number of levels. According to Gilbert *et al.* (2009) neglect is at least as damaging as physical or sexual abuse and we have already noted the links with child fatalities. Ofsted (2014) describe the pervasive and long-term cumulative effect as well documented. Very young children are most at risk of the harmful effects of neglect, but it has also been found to be associated with adolescent suicide and self-harm (Stein *et al.* 2009). Research in recent years has focused on the impact of early neglect on the developing brain, most particularly the development of the hypothalamic-pituitary-adrenal axis, which is involved in self-regulation and emotions. If left unrecognized, this can lead to far-reaching effects on an individual's life chances, including long-term mental health problems and social functioning (Brandon *et al.* 2014).

Practice question

What would you do if you were undertaking a home visit and found a child under the age of 12 years 'home alone'?

Indicators of child neglect

One of the problems in identifying neglect as a form of child maltreatment is that any assessment will be somewhat subjective. The statutory guidance, for instance, uses terminology such as 'adequate' and 'persistent' in its definition. There are likely to be differences of opinion as to the interpretation of these terms and thus differences in agreement between agencies on the threshold for a level of neglect that requires compulsory intervention in family life. A further difficulty is that some of the indicators of neglect may have other causes than the adequacy of parenting, an assessment of which is nevertheless important. A good example of this is developmental delay (Daniel *et al.* 2011).

Judgements are inevitably value laden and based on both personal and professional experiences. Middle-class health professionals can find themselves benchmarking families they meet in the course of their work with their own experiences of child-rearing and child care (i.e. their expectations of parents and parenting are too high). Equally, they can also make somewhat benevolent allowances for struggling or needy parents and thus fail to recognize that the sub-optimal parenting they are witnessing is actually overt neglect of a child. As Brandon *et al.* (2014) suggest, professional training may not help because it encourages student practitioners to value diversity and seek to empower vulnerable parents.

The guidelines produced by the National Institute for Health and Clinical Excellence (NICE) note that there is an ever-present danger that professionals who are working with families with complex problems may use strategies that attempt to empower and support parents/carers, leading to their becoming the primary client, while the risk to the child is accumulating and may go unnoticed (NCCWCH 2009). These concerns were borne out in the review of neglect cases undertaken by Ofsted (2014), which found drift and delay related to inadequate assessments, poor planning and parental non-engagement. Where parents did engage they noted that their needs subsumed those of their children, that they were given too many chances and that children's views, wishes and feelings were not taken into account.

The needs and challenges of keeping focused on the well-being of the child demonstrate how the value of high-quality supervision is critical to good practice. The benefits of supervision are summed up brilliantly by Burton (2009:9) who notes that:

> Supervisors can support critical thinking and reflection, helping practitioners to use both their intuitive and analytic reasoning skills, to value and understand the respective contributions of each, and hopefully to achieve a more integrated approach. Supervision sessions should both support and challenge practitioners, helping them to avoid the temptation to slip uncritically into either an analysis skewed by bias and unfounded assumptions, or simply defaulting to the entrenched 'agency view'.

In helping professionals to recognize and respond to neglect, the NICE guidelines echo the themes of failure or absence in parental care already mentioned. They also recognize the challenges of the contextual elements that underpin this form of child maltreatment. Like Golden *et al.* (2003), there is recognition that parents may not always be aware of the impact of their failures in caring for their children:

> Neglect can be conceptualised as a process involving accumulating risk to the child due to a failure to provide or omission rather than actual incidents of abuse. It is a persistent failure to meet the child's or young person's needs that may or may not be willful.
>
> (NCCWCH 2009:66)

An essential theme of neglect is 'omission' or 'absence of care'. This means that those who practise in settings where there is an ongoing relationship with a family, especially where there is a requirement to undertake home visits, may be best placed to recognize situations where there is neglect of children's health and developmental needs. However, in these situations, there is also the ever-present danger of practitioners becoming accustomed to sub-optimal care, especially where families are living in poor material circumstances where the risk of neglect is, not surprisingly, somewhat greater.

In their classic text, Dingwall *et al.* (1983) refer to the 'rule of optimism' whereby professionals are drawn to find the most positive explanation for what is essentially neglectful parenting. This means that there can be a concomitant failure to recognize and respond to neglect in a timely manner. In all cases, it is the daily lived experiences of the child or young person that should be at the centre of any assessment and referral for concerns about neglect. As the statutory guidance for England notes: 'A desire to think the best of adults and to hope that they can overcome their difficulties should not trump the need to rescue children from chaotic, neglectful and abusive homes' (HM Government 2015a:24).

The importance of benchmarking parental care

In aiming to address the very real difficulties of identifying neglect, as distinct from the effects of material poverty, the NICE guidelines remind practitioners that there is a need to compare what families living with similar constraints manage to achieve against that achieved by families where neglect is an emerging concern. The universality of the contribution of nurses, midwives and health visitors gives unrivalled opportunities to make these comparisons. The guidelines concede that there is 'no diagnostic gold standard' for neglect (p. 68) but that it should be considered or suspected in the situations outlined in Table 7.1.

Table 7.1 Consideration and suspicion of neglect

Neglect should be considered	Neglect should be suspected
• Severe or persistent infestations (e.g. head lice or scabies) • Inappropriate clothing and footwear • Faltering growth (failure to thrive) because of lack of adequate or appropriate diet • Explanation of an injury (e.g. a burn, sunburn or ingestion) that suggests a lack of supervision • The presence of an inappropriate caregiver • A failure to administer essential prescribed treatment for a child • A repeated failure to attend follow-up appointments that are essential for their child's well-being • A failure to engage in the Healthy Child Programme (immunizations, health and development reviews and screening)[1] • A failure, despite access, to obtain NHS treatment for a child's dental care	• Child is persistently smelly and dirty • Poor standard of hygiene that is affecting the child's health • Inadequate provision of food • A living environment that is unsafe for the child's developmental standard • Abandonment of a child • A failure to seek medical advice for a child to the extent that the child's health and well-being is compromised, including ongoing pain

Source: adapted from NCCWCH (2009)

An important finding in the literature on neglect is failure to ensure that children and young people access health care and this is of particular relevance to nurses and midwives and worthy of further analysis at this juncture.

Children who are not brought to appointments: an important feature of neglect

One of the consistent findings in the serious case reviews of children and young people who have died, or been seriously harmed, through child abuse or neglect is that there is a history of missed health care appointments (see e.g. Brandon *et al.* 2009; Wolfe *et al.* 2014). This is also a feature that was found in a more general review that covered all deaths of children aged between 28 days and 18 years over a period of a calendar year (CEMACH 2008). While both documents reflect the fact that death in childhood in the UK is rare (see Chapter 8), they find that there are strong associations with poor social circumstances.

[1]See DH/DSCF 2009a, 2009b.

Health care services have traditionally recorded a failure to attend for out-patient clinic appointments as 'did not attend' or 'DNA' for short. It appears to be common practice for the same process for missed appointments in childhood to be followed as it would be for adults – i.e. a second appointment may be sent, but a further failure to attend results in a letter to the GP (and sometimes to the patient) informing them that no further appointments will be sent unless requested by the GP. While acknowledging that missed appointments are costly to the NHS, and thus the public purse, the issue for children and young people is surely not simply that they *did not attend*, but rather that they *were not brought*.

The problem of missed health care appointments in childhood is raised as a potential child protection concern in the Care Quality Commission (CQC) review of safeguarding children arrangements in the NHS that was published following the death of Peter Connelly (Baby Peter). It is now expected that health services will embed a strategy to address this as part of their safeguarding children policy (CQC 2009). Missing health care appointments can be an important sign that a child is suffering from neglect and may also represent a deteriorating situation within a family, as the extract below from a serious case review illustrates.

Between 1998 and 2008 the children missed a minimum of 129 professional appointments. Undoubtedly, with a family of six children, some of whom had statements of special educational need, there are particular pressures and stresses for parents and a degree of failed appointments would be expected, particularly when the mother was operating as a single parent for periods of time. However, the pattern of failed appointments escalated dramatically during 2007 as relationships with professionals deteriorated. The response to these failures within the agencies was not always actively addressed, or the significance fully understood, and therefore not communicated with partner agencies.

(Birmingham Safeguarding Children Board 2010:10–11)

Powell and Appleton (2012) have argued that a reconceptualization of the common usage of DNA to 'was not brought' (WNB) will better reflect the reality of what happens when a child misses a health care appointment or the family is not in for a home visit. However, there remains more to do to ensure that health care organizations have adequate and appropriate systems in place at the many interfaces between primary and secondary care to both monitor and respond to children's missed appointments (Roe *et al.* 2015).

Nevertheless, it is not just the failure to ensure that children and young people are brought to appointments per se. Neglect of health care can also include a failure to respond to advice from health care professionals once health needs in children are recognized (NCCWCH 2009). In some instances, there may also be 'disguised compliance' (Reder *et al.* 1993) whereby families appear to be addressing issues that may include failed appointments or school attendance, but in reality are continuing to neglect or abuse their child while seeking to appease professionals with what amounts to a 'smokescreen'.

Disguised compliance is a theme that is frequently reported in the serious case review literature alongside other common themes in relation to parental background and difficulties. This means that while practitioners need to ensure that recognition of, and response to, neglect is focused on the child and their daily lived experiences, it is also important to understand the pressures or difficulties that may lead parents to neglect (or otherwise maltreat) their children.

The role of nurses and midwives

This chapter opened by considering the defining attributes of neglect. The focus has been largely at an individual or family level with an emphasis on neglect linked to absences in the provision of parental care and/or supervision. It is important now to take a more positive stance and note that neglect is an issue that is 'ripe' for early help and prevention at a number of levels. The use of a systematic framework to help professionals to objectify neglect and to seek to motivate and work with parents to address deficits is gaining momentum within the safeguarding and child protection field. One example is the work currently being undertaken by the NSPCC on the utility of the Graded Care Profile (Srivastava and Polnay 1997). Another is the Signs of Safety tool.

Signs of Safety

Although principally an intervention used by children's social care workers, the use of the Signs of Safety approach, developed in Australia by Andrew Turnell and Stephen Edwards, is currently being incorporated into provision across the children's workforce in England (Bunn 2013). The approach aims to improve the involvement and buy-in of families and professionals by focusing on family strengths, while also ensuring the safety of the child. The programme draws on solution-focused brief therapy and seeks to support the family in making changes by employing a rating scale to monitor change and ensure that goals are achieved. The structure for this process is provided by a framework for practice that seeks to provide clarity in being open with the family as to what the concerns are (e.g. past harm, future danger); what is working well; what needs to change; and where that change is on a scale of 0–10. Older children are able to reflect their thoughts and experiences via completion of a child-friendly visual image of the framework – i.e. the house of dreams, the house of good things and the house of worries. Proponents of the methodology argue that it improves relationships within the family, job satisfaction of professionals, relationships between parents and professionals, and family involvement in child protection processes.

See: http://www.signsofsafety.net/signs-of-safety/.

Nurses, midwives and health visitors, as universal service providers, have a range of opportunities to address the issue and to ensure that children and young people are protected from the devastating effects of neglect. Health visitors, in particular, have been identified as having a key role in reducing inequalities (NICE 2014b). This can be through the provision of targeted services to children, young people and their parents, or through the delivery of specific programmes such as the Family Nurse Partnership (FNP) outlined in Chapter 2. However, health visitors' preparation for practice and their core role has long since included an expectation that they will develop the broader skills and knowledge that are required to influence policies affecting health. This could ultimately lead to the political imperative to create a society that better prepares and supports parents and the importance of good parenting.

The following case scenarios describe three different presentations of neglect. Links are made to the evidence base for practice and to the statutory guidance. In each case, the actions of the nurse, midwife and health visitor are described in terms of best practice.

Case 1: Jack – a baby at risk of neglect

Jack, a newborn baby, is the third child of Trinity, who is 23 years old. She was 29 weeks' pregnant when she booked for her antenatal care and attended for two of her remaining appointments. Trinity also saw her community midwife, Christina, at home prior to delivering Jack in the maternity unit at 37 weeks, following a precipitate labour. Jack's birth weight was 2.37 kg, he is deemed to be a healthy infant and Trinity is keen to breast feed. Jack is already subject to a child protection plan under the category of 'at risk of neglect'. This resulted from plans that were put in place when Jack was an unborn baby and reflects professionals' concerns about his welfare in the context of his parents' past histories and their somewhat chaotic lifestyles.

The background to Jack's child protection plan is that Trinity's two older children were removed from her care as a result of concerns about the impact of her lifestyle and choice of an unsuitable partner, whose own history of violent and controlling behaviour was believed to put the children at considerable risk. The children, who are now 6 and 7 years of age, had been subject to inconsistent care and extreme physical punishment. They are currently in the long-term care of non-kinship foster parents. Supervised contact between mother and children has been arranged at a local children's centre, but this has not been entirely successful as Trinity has reported difficulty in arranging the transport needed to get her there.

As a child Trinity herself spent periods of time 'in care' after being abandoned by an alcoholic mother, who has since died. Her father, also called Jack, left the family home when Trinity was 2 years old. Contact with him dwindled over time and has now been lost. Trinity failed to reach her potential at school, in part because she was subject to bullying from others due to her somewhat unkempt appearance and poor clothing, but also because she was often absent due to caring for her mother. There has been something of a re-run of her own childhood in recent years: she has experienced an abusive relationship and desertion, poor housing conditions and removal of her children. Trinity has found that strong lager, bought from the local corner shop, has been helpful in numbing the numerous losses and disappointments in her life. As a result of her experiences, she has few friends and finds it difficult to trust professionals.

Jack is the result of a recent relationship with Joel, who works sporadically as a groundsman in the local park. The pregnancy was unplanned. Joel, who is 28 years of age, has three children by two previous partners. He has been rendered homeless as a result of being 'thrown out' by his last partner and has been sleeping in his van. Joel occasionally smokes cannabis, but does not see this as an issue. The couple report that they are keen to make a new life together and to put their past behind them.

Practice point

When faced with overwhelming information and a feeling of helplessness arising from hearing of the difficult background of their clients, such as the removal of previous children in situations of neglect, practitioners and their managers may adopt what Brandon *et al.* (2008) have termed the 'start again syndrome'. This means that they may fail to ensure that the meaning of the past history is incorporated into present-day assessments. This can result in a failure to adequately protect a child, with sometimes tragic results.

It is clear from the time of the late booking that Trinity is a vulnerable young woman who presents as sullen and difficult to engage. Keen to develop a relationship of trust, midwife Christina arranges to see her at home with her partner although there were two 'no access' visits before she was able to gain access. During the home visit Christina discovers more about the context of the removal of Trinity's two previous children, her violent relationship with their father and her lack of family and social support. During the visit Joel is watchful and silent, as he would be during any contact that Christina has with the family in the coming months. The housing conditions appear to be poor – a small dark room in a privately rented house. Although she feels sorry for Trinity, Christina considers that there are clear risks to the unborn baby arising from the maternal history, the past history of neglect, the removal of two previous children, the substance misuse and the poor engagement of both partners. These concerns are compounded by the late presentation for booking, the missed appointments and the no access visits. In addition, during the home visit Christina sees little in the way of preparedness for a baby. A further concern is the newness of the couple's relationship and the fact that very little information is gleaned in terms of Joel's previous family and social history or the whereabouts of his three children. Fleetingly, Christina also senses an element of quiet control from Joel that she thinks may be an indicator of the possibility of domestic violence or abuse (Lombard and Macmillan 2013).

Christina informs the couple that she will be discussing their case with a senior midwife and that she will also be asking children's social care to consider undertaking a more detailed assessment and programme of support. The reasons for her concerns are shared with the couple. There is a passive acceptance of this proposed action and a referral to social care is progressed.

> ## Pre-birth child protection conferences and reviews
>
> Where an assessment under Section 47 of the Children Act 1989 gives rise to concerns that an unborn child may be likely to suffer significant harm, local authority children's social care may decide to convene an ICPC prior to the child's birth (HM Government 2015a). Such a conference should have the same status, and proceed in the same way, as other ICPCs, including decisions about a child protection plan for the unborn child. The involvement of midwifery services is vital in such cases.

The named midwife

Christina sought supervision in relation to the safeguarding aspects of the case with the named midwife for safeguarding children. According to the statutory guidance, all providers of maternity services are expected to have a named midwife, in addition to the named nurse and named doctor roles (HM Government 2015a).

Case 1 continued

Following the ICPC, Christina becomes a member of the core group, which works with the family to promote parenting strengths and reduce the risk of neglect. This includes encouraging the couple to engage with professionals and to plan for the safe parenting of Jack. In doing so, Christina works closely with the allocated social worker, including undertaking a joint home visit shortly after Jack's arrival. Christina also ensures that she provides a detailed handover to the health visiting team who will care for the family once they are discharged from midwifery care.

One of the key issues facing the family is that of housing. After her older children were placed in care, and with the threat of serious domestic abuse from her previous partner, Trinity became temporarily homeless. Poor housing is recognized to be a factor in social exclusion and to present a safeguarding risk to children (including risk of accidents and fire). Housing services, as a function of the local authority, are bound by similar statutory duties to health services in relation to their safeguarding and child protection responsibilities. Housing has a particular responsibility to take action with landlords to improve conditions when they are likely to have an impact on the health and safety of vulnerable occupants, including children (HM Government 2015a). Thus, an early action is to review the housing needs for the newly formed family. Only time will tell if the child protection plan has been successful in protecting Jack by monitoring his welfare and providing additional support for his parents.

Markers of good practice: the role of the midwife

Christina recognizes the risk factors for neglect of the unborn baby and helps to ensure a timely and proactive response. She seeks supervision from the named midwife and follows up her telephone referral to children's social care in writing.

Christina is able to play a leading role in the core group who are responsible for ensuring that the requirements of the child protection plan are met.

Although she feels sorry for Trinity, Christina keeps a focus on the need to safeguard and promote the welfare of the child. She is open and honest with the parents as to the reasons for her concerns, informs them of the referral to children's social care and is prepared to offer some flexibility to meet their needs.

Christina ensures that the health visitor has a detailed handover before she discharges the family from her care.

Case 2: Courtney and Kendra – faltering growth

Courtney and Kendra are the 18-month-old twin children of Maxine and Declan, who originate from the Irish travelling community. They are their first-born children. The twins have been subject to a child protection plan, under the category of neglect, for a period of 9 months, as there have been concerns that they were malnourished and poorly cared for. The ICPC was followed 3 months later by a review child protection conference (RCPC), and a second review conference has been arranged to take place 6 months after this one. This is in keeping with *Working Together* which sets the parameters for the timing of the initial and subsequent review conferences (HM Government 2015a:47).

Amanda, the health visitor, is a key member of the core group and has been working closely with Maxine and Declan, children's social care, a family centre worker and a Home-Start volunteer to ensure that the children's needs are met, and that they do not suffer additional harm. She has also been liaising with other health professionals involved with the family, including the GP, community paediatrician and dietician. Amanda arranges for a nursery nurse from the children and family team to provide support and advice on play and activities for the twins. The additional support that has been provided for the family appears to have led to a much improved situation for Courtney and Kendra. Although they remain small, they now appear to be thriving and are reaching their expected developmental milestones. Indeed, with a vocabulary of around 80–100 words and a number of two-word sentences, Kendra appears to be above average in her speech and language development. Although there were initial difficulties in engaging the parents with the objectives of the child protection plan, they are now appreciating the difference that it has made for the family.

The events that led to the child protection plan began when the children were aged 9 months and concerns were raised via an anonymous call to children's social care saying that the children were not being fed properly. In the first instance Amanda was asked if she would agree to making an assessment and to weigh the infants. She had not visited the family since the twins were around 4 months old, at which time Declan's mother had been staying and all had appeared to be satisfactory. A review of the twins was somewhat overdue. However, when Amanda called, there was 'no reply' despite the fact that this was an arranged visit. She left a card, and then tried to call, but the mobile telephone number that she had been given previously was unobtainable. A couple of days later Amanda called by on an unannounced visit. This time the door was opened by Declan, who said that the babies were asleep and that it was not convenient to call. He added that it was a bad time for them as he had just lost his job. Given that the initial concerns had been raised by children's social care, Amanda reported back to them and a joint visit was arranged.

At this visit the parents were informed that a call had been received concerning the welfare of the children. Both professionals were also concerned to find indications of neglectful care. In respect of the infants' weight, Amanda found that their initial weight gain had tailed off. When plotted on a centile chart, she noted that it had crossed from the 25th to below the 3rd centile, suggesting faltering growth. While it was accepted that the twins were small for their age due to their prematurity and genetic make-up, the current weights, taken in context with other indicators of neglect, were a cause of concern (NCCWCH 2009). In addition to the faltering growth, there were other factors of note. These included the fact that Kendra presented with an excoriating nappy rash and that both infants looked somewhat grubby and pale, with dark shadows under their eyes. When Amanda and the social worker arrived at the house, they were also concerned to find that Courtney was strapped into a buggy, while Kendra was asleep on the sofa. Declan and Maxine had recently become the owners of a puppy, who was in the stages of being 'house-trained'. Both parents presented as 'flat' and somewhat apathetic to the needs of the babies and their new pet. The house was extremely untidy, with piles of damp washing draped over the furniture. Declan explained that his mother had returned to Ireland and that they had not parted in good company, mainly because of the tensions between Maxine and her mother-in-law. The couple also admitted that they had missed an immunization appointment for the twins.

Referral was made via the GP for a paediatric assessment, as it was important to be clear as to the possible cause of the faltering growth. The health visitor also asked the parents to complete a 'food diary' for the twins and arranged a follow-up visit a week later. The key concern was of neglect and that these were unsupported young parents who were struggling with a range of issues, including estrangement from their wider network of family and recent unemployment. There had also been a pattern of neighbour disputes on the new estate where the family were living. Unfortunately, the parents did not comply with the advice to complete the diary, neither did they take the children to the appointment with the paediatrician. As a result of this, Section 47 enquiries were initiated by children's social care, an ICPC was held and the twins were made subject to a child protection plan. The parents attended the conference, and accepted the need for a period of intensive help and monitoring to ensure the well-being of their babies.

Practice question

If you were the health visitor for this family what could you be expected to contribute to the child protection plan?

The review child protection conference

There is a constant flux in the numbers and names of children and young people who are subject to a child protection plan, with most plans in place for between 3 and 12 months. The purpose of the RCPC is to reconvene a meeting between parents and professionals (children too, where they are of an age to contribute) to review the health and developmental progress of the child/children against the outcomes set out in the child protection plan, amending the plan if necessary. Importantly, it is the point at which an inter-agency decision can be made as to whether or not the plan can be discontinued, and if so, what ongoing support may be needed, including the possibility of 'stepping down' to a Children Act 1989 Section 17 'child in need' plan.

In order for a child protection plan to be discontinued one of the following must apply:

- It is judged that the child is no longer continuing to, or is likely to, suffer significant harm and therefore no longer requires safeguarding by means of a child protection plan;
- the child and family have moved to another area. In such cases the receiving local authority should convene a child protection conference within 15 days of being notified of the move. [...]

- the child has reached the age of 18 years (to end the child protection plan, the local authority should have a review around the child's birthday and this should be planned in advance), has died or has permanently left the United Kingdom.

(HM Government 2015a:49)

Case 2 continued

Kendra and Courtney have been subject to a child protection plan in the category of 'neglect' for 9 months. During this period of time there has been an intensive package of multi-agency work with the family. Amanda, the health visitor, plays a key role in ensuring that the children receive their immunizations, attend appointments with the GP, paediatrician and dietician and that these health professionals are aware of the child protection status of the twins. She also plans and supervises the nursery nurse input, which has helped to ensure that Maxine and Declan engage in play activities that support the children's development. Amanda works closely with the allocated social worker to monitor the twins' health and well-being. There are now signs of both improved physical care and pattern of growth. Importantly, the parents have complied with the interventions, and Declan has recently found work. Amanda is anticipating that the outcome of the RCPC will be an inter-agency decision to discontinue the child protection plan.

Practice question

If you were the health visitor attending the conference what evidence might you present to persuade colleagues that the children are no longer at risk of significant harm? What would you be able to contribute to ongoing care to ensure that the children are safeguarded in the future?

This case has provided a 'window' on the processes by which children and young people can be protected from harm. A marker of the success of the child protection process is to consider the numbers of re-referrals back into the system, and while the overall numbers of children on a plan have increased, the percentage of re-referrals has decreased steadily over the past 5 years (DfE 2014a).

Child's perspective

The provision of timely intervention and a plan that was centred on the children's well-being has helped to ensure that the twins achieve their health and developmental outcomes. Having a plan in place for children who are suffering from neglect has been found to support proactive action to improve their safety and well-being. It will be important to review the children on a regular basis as part of any 'step-down' plan to ensure that progress is maintained.

Markers of good practice: the role of the health visitor

Amanda works collaboratively with all those involved in addressing the safeguarding children issues. Her expert knowledge of infant feeding, child health and child development underpins the relationship with other stakeholders, including the parents.

Although children's social care took the statutory lead in managing the child protection aspects, Amanda is a lynchpin in terms of liaising with other health professionals (GP, paediatrician, dietician) and in supporting a nursery nurse in the provision of a programme of play and activities that has been rewarding to both the twins and their parents.

Amanda carefully documents her assessment and produces written reports which she presents at core group and RCPCs. These are shared with the parents in advance of these meetings.

In recognizing the intensity of the relationship with this family, and her feelings of distress at the initial visits, Amanda seeks supervision with her allocated supervisor, and additional support from the named nurse safeguarding children.

Amanda completes clear, contemporaneous records of the events and her actions (NMC 2015).

Case 3: Logan – an accidental ingestion

Logan is an active and inquisitive 4-year-old, who spends alternate week-ends with his father, Charlie. The pair have a great deal of fun together and Logan looks forward to the visits. Logan's parents separated when he was 18 months of age. Charlie's substance misuse and addiction was a feature of the ending of their relationship. However, he agreed to attend the local substance misuse service for treatment and being 'clean' is a condition of the courts for his contact time with his son. As part of his treatment, Charlie has been prescribed suboxone (buprenorphine and naloxone), which after an initial requirement to 'consume on premises', he now has dispensed on a weekly basis. This new regime has marked a sustained period of compliance and stability with his treatment.

After a day out at the local zoo, Logan is rather fractious and tired. As a treat, Charlie allows Logan to have a nap in his bedroom. Unfortunately, he has failed to remember that his packet of suboxone is on the bedside cabinet. A short while later he finds that Logan has opened the box and that there are a number of tablets missing. Searching frantically he finds one nibbled tablet on the floor, and half a tablet on the bedcover. Logan is difficult to rouse and is breathing slowly, but noisily. An ambulance is called. Later that day Logan is transferred from the local hospital to the paediatric intensive care unit (PICU) for respiratory support and monitoring. Thankfully, he makes a full recovery.

With support from the hospital's liaison health visitor, PICU staff contact the local children's social care department. A multi-agency strategy discussion, chaired by a senior social worker and involving hospital and community health professionals and the police, is held. While it is accepted that this was an accidental overdose, the need to guard against future risk is clear. The case will progress to a Section 47 enquiry and an ICPC. The local community provider of substance misuse services will also raise the event as a 'serious incident'.

The adverse effects of accidental exposure to buprenorphine in young children

A paper by Geib *et al.* (2006) reports on five cases of toddlers with life-threatening respiratory and mental status depression after accidental ingestion of buprenorphine. This series included children who accessed parental, other relatives' and a family friend's medication. The authors note that sublingual absorption may lead to significant toxicity in small children by merely placing the medication in their mouths. They recommend that parents in homes where buprenorphine is used should be warned of the risks of paediatric exposure.

 Child's perspective

Logan has ingested a potentially lethal dose of a dangerous medication. He required intensive care – a frightening and bewildering experience for any individual, especially a young child. Once he recovers, he is likely to experience the additional pressures and reprisals that this incident adds to his parents' already difficult relationship.

Case 3 continued

As part of the response to this serious incident, Molly, a substance misuse practitioner, is asked by her manager to work with the local safeguarding children lead to see if there are lessons that can be learned. This request was made under the auspices of the Serious Incident Framework (NHS England 2015). One of the issues raised in the subsequent investigation is the degree to which Charlie's care coordinator considered the implications of the treatment in relation to his contact with Logan (or indeed any other children).

Molly concludes that the way in which the service worked to 'protect' the privacy and confidentiality of their clients, including keeping separate sets of records, led to failures in recording the details of any child care responsibilities, as well as proactive liaison with other agencies. This appears to be contrary to best practice (Cleaver *et al.* 2008).

Molly and her safeguarding lead approach the LSCB with a proposal to draw up a protocol to improve joint working. Furthermore, the service's care pathway for the treatment and management of opioid addiction is revised to include more explicit detail on the importance of educating clients and their families about the dangers of accidental ingestion of medication by young children (NICE 2007). Client records are also redesigned to ensure that details of family members, including dependent children, are completed even where they are not members of the same household.

> ## Markers of good practice: the role of the substance misuse practitioner
>
> Molly works jointly with the safeguarding children lead to review this serious incident and consider the learning from it (NHS England 2015).
>
> Improvements are made to the process of care planning and assessment to ensure that the needs of children (and risks to them) will become an integral part of the care delivered by the service.
>
> Molly seeks to underpin her review with the evidence base for good practice.

Summary

This chapter has considered neglect as a form of child maltreatment. Neglect is seen as an 'omission' of care that can be deliberate, but more commonly occurs as a result of a range of parental difficulties. The impact of neglect can be as serious as other forms of child maltreatment, including the potential to contribute to the death of a child. Despite the wealth of published evidence on the harmful effects of neglect, an informed and authoritative response to child neglect remains somewhat elusive (Brandon *et al* 2014b; Ofsted 2014).

Failure to attend for health care is an important indicator of neglect and robust systems need to be in place to ensure that children who are not brought to appointments are followed up. The three cases that have been presented are drawn from the realities of practice. The first case introduced Trinity, Joel and baby Jack. The past history of the parents and their current lifestyle carry a recognized risk of neglect. The second case considered malnutrition and other factors as indicative of the neglect of twins, Courtney and Kendra. An RCPC considered whether or not the plan could be discontinued. Finally, a serious incident concerning a young child's accidental ingestion of a prescribed semi-synthetic opioid, with a potentially tragic outcome, was discussed. A community midwife, a health visitor and a substance misuse practitioner were the key professionals involved in the cases. These fictional cases have been portrayed in a realistic way, but the aim here is to demonstrate how easy it can be to 'feel sorry' for the parents. However, the over-arching message, that the daily lived experience of the child is the most important factor in any assessment, is clear.

Key points

- Neglect is the most common reason for children and young people to have a child protection plan.

- An essential theme of neglect is 'omission' or 'absence of care'; the effects are cumulative.

- Neglect can lead to serious outcomes for children and young people, including fatality. It co-exists with other forms of abuse.

- When children do not attend health appointments this should be conceived as 'was not brought' rather than 'did not attend'.

- Professionals working with neglectful families need to ensure that they access high-quality supervision that will both support and challenge their thinking.

8

Child death and serious case reviews

Learning outcomes

This chapter will help you to:

- Be aware of the purpose and function of a serious case review and how the learning from these reviews contributes to improvements in safeguarding and child protection practice.
- Understand the purpose and function of statutory child death review processes (child death overview panel and the rapid response).
- Appreciate the role that child death review has in the prevention of future child deaths.
- Gain insight into the role of the designated nurse (and doctor).

Introduction

This chapter aims to help nurses, midwives and health visitors to gain an appreciation of statutory LSCB case review procedures that are set out in Chapters 4 and 5 of *Working Together* (HM Government 2015a). The chapter essentially has two parts: the first part centres on the serious case review (SCR) process and the second part on child death reviews. The well-established process of SCR follows the rare cases of child maltreatment-related deaths and serious child care incidents, while the more recently introduced child death review processes apply in all cases of child death – expected and unexpected. In the case of unexpected death, a process called the 'rapid response', which involves professionals from health, social care and the police is enacted and this is also outlined. Contribution to SCRs and child death review processes are a key component of the roles and responsibilities of designated and named nurses and their teams, but any nurse, midwife or health visitor could potentially contribute to these reviews as the front-line practitioner involved with the care of the child or family.

Two cases are discussed. The first is the death of a teenager, HH, who died from a treatable medical condition in the context of neglect. Unlike all the other scenarios in this book, this is an actual case that was subject to SCR, although, as is usual practice, the child is not named in the review (Herefordshire

Safeguarding Children Board 2014). The second case concerns Tegan, who has died unexpectedly at the age of 11 weeks. The circumstances of her death, the process of rapid response and the child death review process are outlined.

The death of an infant, child or young person, whether expected or sudden and unexpected, with or without suspicious circumstances, is a tragedy for all those involved. In the UK today, as in all developed countries, death in childhood is, thankfully, rare. Because of this, when a child dies there may be a resultant groundswell of action that is concerned with ensuring that lessons are learned or changes made to prevent future child deaths. In many cases, such action is led by the bereaved family and friends. This would include actions taken to gain meaning and to help to prevent such deaths in the future. Examples here may well include activity following the deaths of children from cancer, road traffic collisions or the deaths of young people from suicide or self-harm. Child death review processes garner actions of parents, professionals, wider communities and governments to help to learn lessons and make changes to prevent future deaths.

When a child or young person has died or is seriously injured, and abuse or neglect are recognized to have contributed, the circumstances of the case will always be reviewed in some depth to see if lessons can be learned. A minority of child maltreatment deaths will become high profile. In these cases, the public and politicians may also demand action and, caught up with the horror of these deaths, there may be what can only be described as gratuitous vilification of professionals (e.g. in the cases of Victoria Climbié, Peter Connelly, Khyra Ishaq and Daniel Pelka). The effect of this can be devastating, with an ever-present danger that practitioners from the range of agencies who contribute to child protection and safeguarding (i.e. professionals from health, early years, education, children's social care and the police service) will fail to engage in this work, be this at the front line or as a chosen specialty later in their careers. This in turn raises a risk of jeopardizing the safety and well-being of a generation of children, young people and their families.

Responses to the death of a child, however caused, must be supportive, proportionate and timely, while maximizing opportunities for improvements in knowledge, professional practice and policies for children, young people and their families. In recognizing both the unusualness of death in childhood, as well as the impact of policy on the broader welfare of children, young people and their families, Jenny and Isaac (2006:265) note that 'The death of a child is a sentinel event in a community, and a defining marker of a society's policies of safety and health.'

Developing an understanding of SCR and child death review processes aims to assist readers in making the links between preventative action and policies that promote children and young people's safety and health. As such, it will help to strengthen and consolidate the learning and improvement in safeguarding and child protection that this book aims to promote. The knowledge gained may in turn support nurses and midwives in making practical and positive contributions to improvements in safeguarding and promoting the welfare of children, young people and their families in the future.

Serious case reviews

The process for undertaking SCRs is set out in Chapter 4 of *Working Together* and is part of the requirements for the establishment of local learning and improvement frameworks to both share good practice and to learn from cases that 'go wrong' (HM Government 2015a:72).[1] SCRs are thus statutory processes that are commissioned by the chair of the LSCB in cases of serious child maltreatment. Some 2 per cent of all child deaths result in an SCR (DfE 2014b). This includes cases where abuse or neglect of a child is known or suspected and either the child dies, or is seriously harmed and there are concerns about organizations or professionals that have worked together to safeguard the child. An independent reviewer will be appointed to lead the process and author the SCR report.

Importantly, an SCR is not an investigation into how a child died or who was responsible. These are issues that the coroner and criminal courts will determine. SCRs are also not part of any disciplinary enquiry into an individual's practice; poor practice would be a matter for the employing organization to address through their internal procedures.

As detailed in the guidance, LSCBs will always conduct an SCR when a child dies (including by suspected suicide) and abuse or neglect are known or suspected to be a factor. This may include situations where a child has been killed by a mentally ill parent or carer, or where substance misuse or domestic violence are known to be present. LSCBs may also commission an SCR when a child has been seriously harmed and it is thought that there may be lessons to be learned about the way in which local services worked together. This would include cases involving children who have received life-threatening injuries or permanent impairment or following serious sexual abuse, when a parent has been murdered, or where a child has been harmed following a serious assault perpetrated by another child or an adult. Some, but by no means all, cases will already be known to children's social care or other targeted or specialist services and a minority of the children subject to review may have been subject to a child protection plan (Brandon *et al.* 2014a). Given the universality of health care services, it would be extremely unusual if the child and their family were not known to health care professionals. This means that health services (and for school-age children, education providers) are key contributors to the reviews, perhaps by being interviewed by a report author or by taking part in a learning event with other practitioners and agencies. Contributing to an SCR is an opportunity to ensure that the 'child's story' is told, that good practice is shared and that any learning for the future is identified. SCRs are not about apportioning blame, and they should seek to reflect the practice situation at the time, not with the benefit of hindsight (an issue that the media do not always grasp). Munro (2011:43) helpfully makes reference to the fact that 'Harm can never be totally prevented. Risk decisions should, therefore, be judged by the quality of the decision-making, not by the outcome.'

[1]see Vincent (2009) for a review of similar reports across the UK.

Practice point

In cases that may progress to an SCR practitioners may be asked to hand their records to their safeguarding lead. This is known as 'securing records' and its purpose is to guard against loss or interference and to allow the organization to begin to draw up chronologies of its involvement with the child and family. It does not indicate mistrust of front-line practitioners.

LSCBs usually have a multi-agency SCR subcommittee that aids the decision-making of the LSCB chair as to whether or not an SCR should be undertaken. Advice can also be taken from another LSCB chair or from the government's national panel of independent experts who have been established to provide support for the SCR process (DfE 2014b). In its first year of operation, this panel oversaw the initiation of 184 SCRs in England, and debated the non-initiation of a further 66 reviews. Health services are normally represented on the SCR subcommittee through their commissioning organization. In most cases the representative will be the designated nurse and/or designated doctor for safeguarding children.

SCRs should generally be completed within 6 months. The process and content of the final report is guided by the terms of reference negotiated by the LSCB chair and SCR subcommittee. The guidance notes that any learning model that is consistent with the principles of independence, proportionality and transparency can be used to inform the structure and format of the review. Systems methodology, a layered approach that reflects the context for the delivery of care, is recommended (HM Government 2015a). Practitioners, managers and families (including the child/surviving children) should be involved in contributing to the review. A report of the SCR, and the response of the LSCB to the report, must be written in plain English and published. Publication is on the LSCB website, where the report has to remain readily accessible for a minimum of 12 months, and be available on request after that. It may also be published on the SCR online repository set up and managed by the Association of Independent LSCB Chairs and the NSPCC. The NSPCC also provide periodic themed briefings of learning from SCRs, and many of these will be of interest to nurses and midwives (see below).

Activity

Visit your LSCB website. Are there any SCR reports available to download? If so, read a report and reflect on the meaning of the findings and recommendations for your own practice and that of your colleagues. Alternatively, visit the national repository and select a report to read and consider.
    See: http://www.lscbChairs.org.uk/SCR_repository.

Action plans

SCRs should aim to contribute to learning and improvement of safeguarding and child protection practice at a local level. Action plans are therefore a key component of the review, as they set out a framework for taking forward the recommendations and a means of apportioning accountability and monitoring progress. There will be recommendations for single agencies, as well as recommendations that aim to improve inter-agency working. An example of the layout of an action plan is illustrated in Table 8.1.

Implementation of recommendations arising from SCRs can take up to two years, depending on their complexity and the capacity of individuals and agencies to make changes. In my experience it is important to be realistic and also to limit single and multi-agency recommendations to between four and six proposals.

Learning for health professionals

The NSPCC have usefully summarized the learning from SCRs for the health sector,[2] with particular emphasis on those working in emergency departments (EDs) and paediatric services. The briefing includes reference to a number of key issues that they identified as themes from a number of reviews. The learning points are highlighted in the box below and readers are encouraged to think about how these might be addressed to improve practice by completing the second column.

Learning point	How might practice be improved?
Attendances at the emergency department were seen as incidents in isolation, rather than as part of a bigger picture	
The child or young person was not brought to their health care appointments	
Health professionals had difficulty in working with those from other agencies	
Assessment focused on the physical health needs of the child (i.e. was not holistic)	
Assessment and care was heavily influenced by assertive parents	
The risks to children were not assessed when treating parents/siblings	
There was a lack of assessment of safeguarding and child protection needs for 16- and 17-year-olds (especially for risk of child sexual exploitation)	

[2]http://www.nspcc.org.uk/preventing-abuse/child-protection-system/case-reviews/learning/health/.

Table 8.1 SCR action plan

Recommendations	Action	Evidence	Outcome	Lead officer	Date for completion	Progress (RAG)
These will reflect the recommendations outlined in the report	Action needed to achieve the recommendations Needs to be: *SMART* Specific Measureable Achievable Realistic Timely	How will you provide assurance that the action has been completed? For example, a new policy or copies of meeting notes	How this action will improve services to children and families and better safeguard and protect children	Name or designation of person responsible	For example, 6 months after publication of the report	This column will be used to monitor progress on an agreed 'RAG' (i.e. red, amber, green) rating

Research into learning lessons from SCRs reflects the importance of ensuring that practitioners who find themselves drawn into the process are adequately supported and provided with feedback in terms of lessons learned (Sidebotham *et al.* 2010). While those who took part in the study agreed that SCRs were not about apportioning blame, they generally stated that this should not detract from ensuring accountability for practice. Contributing to, or indeed authoring a serious case review, can be a stressful experience and it is important that feedback and the opportunity to debrief are offered. The final section of this part of the chapter considers an example of an SCR and demonstrates how the learning can feed into improvements in practice.

Case 1: SCR of child HH

Child HH was a 17-year-old male, originally from Poland, whose tragic and untimely death from diabetic ketoacidosis (DKA) occurred in the context of severe neglect. The circumstances surrounding the death met the criteria for an SCR (Herefordshire Safeguarding Children Board 2014). In summary, HH was known to children's social care services as a looked-after child following a number of difficulties, including abandonment by his mother who was reported to be suffering from mental health problems and not consistently providing food or warmth for her children. At the time of his death, HH was living apart from his family in supported housing. He was not in education, employment or training (NEET) and had been known to the police and youth offending service. Following his diagnosis some 16 months previously, HH had shown only partial compliance with the treatment and monitoring of his condition, a factor that was exacerbated by inadequacies in the provision of his care. The SCR makes for interesting reading and cogent links are made with the evidence base for practice throughout. The author considers individual practice issues, but also references cultural, structural and organizational dimensions. These include a failure to follow protocols for hospital admission of 16- and 17-year-olds, poor use of information systems, management vacancies and practitioner sick leave. Crucially, HH was not always seen as a child and his voice and wishes were not consistently sought (or heard). The report contains a number of specific learning points for health services. These relate to:

- the provision of CAMHS support for children and young people facing a diagnosis of a long-term condition;
- ensuring that 16- and 17-year-olds are seen as children and any safeguarding or child protection issues identified;
- the following of WNB protocols for children not attending their appointments;
- improving information-sharing and communication across the interface of health service provision and with other agencies;

- supporting non-health colleagues in their understanding of the meaning of an enduring health problem;
- not using family members as interpreters;
- ensuring child protection supervision and support is made available and accessible to those working in adult health services.

Practice question

Fong (2014) has suggested that 'ideologies of adolescence may be set by a discourse of delinquency and not by poor health'. How can young people's competence in taking responsibility for the management of their long-term condition be assessed, supported and evaluated?

Child death review processes

While there have been significant improvements in childhood mortality rates over the years, the UK has higher rates of child deaths when compared with other European countries. This is particularly the case for infant mortality and for children who are suffering from chronic health conditions. Marked social inequalities are also apparent (Wolfe *et al.* 2014). Statutory child death review processes have been a requirement for LSCBs in England since April 2008 and the details of what is required are set out in Chapter 5 of *Working Together* (HM Government 2015a). These standardized processes and procedures build on the experiences and learning from other countries (most notably the USA) as well as various 'early starter' panels (Sidebotham *et al.* 2008, 2011) and regional systems in the UK (CEMACH 2008). The primary purpose of child death reviews is to seek to understand why children die and whether there are 'modifiable factors' that may lead to local or national initiatives to reduce the risk of future deaths. The aggregated findings from all child deaths should be used to inform local strategic planning as well as any regional and national initiatives to prevent child deaths. As such, child death review processes are primarily a public health function.

Although the majority of child deaths are reported to be 'entirely non-suspicious' (Fox 2008), the child death review process provides an additional opportunity for inter-agency consideration of the possibility of maltreatment as a contributory factor in the death. This function addresses long-standing concerns in the UK and elsewhere that there may be under-ascertainment of such deaths and vilification of some bereaved parents. Baroness Kennedy's working group on sudden unexpected death in infancy (SUDI) sought to address these issues through systematic enquiry and improvements in the evidence base (RCP/RCPCH 2004). The so-called 'Kennedy principles' continue to inform review processes (HM Government 2015a). As we have noted elsewhere in this book, although child maltreatment deaths are usually perceived to take place as a result of inflicted physical injury or severe neglect, deaths of children and young people may also occur within the context of historical or long-standing maltreatment, including emotional and sexual abuse (Davies and Ward 2012; Brandon *et al.* 2014; Wolfe *et al.* 2014). Child death review processes thus provide opportunities to improve safeguarding practice, to prevent future child deaths and to impact more widely on the health and well-being of children, young people and their families.

The guidance upholds an expectation that all LSCBs in England will ensure that there are procedures in place to support a multi-agency 'rapid response' to unexpected deaths and that all childhood deaths occurring within a local authority area will be reviewed at a child death overview panel (CDOP). The stated purposes of these processes are to identify:

- any cases that may require further investigation, including the need for a serious case review;
- any concern about the health and safety of children in the area;
- any wider public health or safety concerns that arise from a particular death, or pattern of deaths in the area.

The processes are now considered in more detail.

The child death overview panel

The CDOP, which is made up of senior leads from a range of agencies, is responsible for reviewing all deaths of children (up to the age of 18 years, excluding stillborn babies and planned lawful terminations) who live within a local authority area (or areas) served by an LSCB. They will collect and collate information on each child, seeking relevant information from professionals and, where appropriate, family members. The panel will meet to discuss each case, determine if the death was preventable (or not) and whether there are any modifiable factors that contributed to the death. They will also suggest actions or recommendations to prevent such deaths in the future.

Preventable child deaths

[Deaths] in which modifiable factors may have contributed to the death. These are factors defined as those, where, if actions could be taken through national or local initiatives, the risk of future child deaths could be reduced.

(HM Government 2015a:85)

CDOP findings are reported back to the LSCB. If there are suspicions that neglect or abuse was a contributing factor in the child's death, the CDOP can also refer the case back to the LSCB chair for consideration of an SCR (if one is not already in place).

Practice point

All deaths of children and young people should be notified to the local designated person who coordinates the CDOP process. Health professionals should have access to the national forms for making such reports (see HM Government, 2015a:82) and know how the process operates in their locality. It is important to remember to ensure that children and young people who die at home are notified to the designated person.

Local CDOPs usually have a fixed core multi-disciplinary membership drawn from the key agencies who are represented at the LSCB, with others co-opted as necessary (e.g. a road traffic officer if a road traffic collision death is being reviewed). Public health and child health professionals will be core members of the panel. A typical panel and its functions is outlined in Table 8.2.

Table 8.2 Role and function of CDOP members

Role	Function
Chair	Acts as the LSCB chair's representative
Public health consultant	Will contribute specialist public health advice on trends, statistics, demography, health protection and prevention
Specialist community public health nurse/designated nurse safeguarding children	Advice on health care matters (including prevention), child development, specialist safeguarding children knowledge, relevant case information, including bereavement support
Designated paediatrician for unexpected child deaths	Advice on pathology, post-mortem results, treatment regimes, relevant case information
Senior manager, children's social care	Advice on child care and safeguarding issues, relevant case information
Senior ambulance officer	Relevant case information and advice on emergency response
Senior manager, education	Advice on education matters, relevant case information
Senior police officer	Advice on criminal and public safety aspects, relevant case information
Co-opted members (e.g. midwife, neonatologist, pathologist, road traffic officer, hospice nurse)	Will attend according to the nature of the deaths being discussed to provide an expert opinion

Involvement of parents

The Lullaby Trust (formerly known as the Foundation for the Study of Infant Deaths) has produced an excellent leaflet called *Child Death Review: A Guide for Parents and Carers* (Lullaby Trust 2013) that can be ordered as a hard copy or downloaded from their website.[3] This leaflet, which should be made readily available to all bereaved parents, also serves as a useful introduction to child death review for health professionals.

In essence, when a child dies, the parents should be informed that their child's death will be reviewed by a CDOP. Where the death of a child is unexpected, the rapid response process has a number of points of direct contact with families and there is anecdotal and research-based evidence that parents find this helpful. Parents should be assured that the key objective of the CDOP is to learn lessons that may help to improve the health, safety and well-being of children and to prevent future deaths. Although it is not appropriate for parents to attend panel meetings, they are encouraged to contribute any comments or questions they might have to the review and the panel will need to ensure that feedback is provided accordingly. As noted at the outset, taking action and learning lessons from the tragedy of child death may help parents, families, professionals and communities to address the terrible loss of a child and find some meaning in being able to better protect the health, safety and well-being of others.

Rapid response

The rapid response to unexpected deaths in childhood is best described as an inter-agency approach that seeks to gather information to help in determining why a child died and to better support the family. The key agencies involved are health and the police, although there is also a role for children's social care and other agencies who may have been involved with the child or their family. CCGs are required to appoint a designated paediatrician for unexpected deaths in childhood who will take an overall lead on rapid response, including offering support and expertise to on-call paediatricians as required. Unexpected deaths in childhood are defined as:

> the death of an infant or child which was not anticipated as a significant possibility for example, 24 hours before the death; or where there was an unexpected collapse or incident leading to or precipitating the vents which led to the death.
>
> (HM Government 2015a:85)

Access your LSCB rapid response protocol so that you are aware of how this system operates in your area. Find out who holds responsibility for the role of designated doctor for unexpected deaths and who takes the role of the senior health care professional in joint home (or place of death) visits.

[3]http://www.lullabytrust.org.uk/file/-----internal-documents/Lullaby-CDR_Booklet.pdf.

The immediate response

The immediate response to a child's unexpected collapse or death will normally involve ambulance transport of the child to an ED, with ongoing attempts at resuscitation, if appropriate. Even where it appears as though the child may have been dead for some time, it is considered best practice to take the body to an ED, rather than straight to a mortuary. This will enable any chance of successful resuscitation, help to ensure early expert examination of the child's body by a paediatrician and facilitate the collection of samples and specimens in accordance with legislation and guidance (RCP/RCPCH 2004).

Clearly, the ED is also an environment where nursing staff are on hand to offer first-line bereavement support to parents, often in conjunction with a faith leader. Nursing staff who are allocated to care for parents at this time should ensure that the parents are given an opportunity to hold and spend time with their child, while they keep a discreet presence. Staff may also offer parents a memento, such as a lock of hair or footprint from their child.

In some cases – for example accidental deaths of older children or in order to preserve a crime scene – transfer to an ED may not be possible. However, as in all cases of unexpected death in childhood, the key aspects of rapid response, such as inter-agency communication, information-sharing and planning, should still occur.

The police are involved in all unexpected deaths. Once the death of a child is confirmed, a comprehensive health and social history will be gathered jointly by the police and a paediatrician while the family is in the ED. This is done primarily to help to ascertain the cause of death and to identify any suspicious indicators. The coroner is also informed of the death, and from this point onwards will have jurisdiction over the body.

The initial information-sharing and planning meeting/discussion

The paediatrician (either on-call or designated) will initiate an information-sharing and planning meeting between lead agencies (health, police and social care) and others who may have been involved in the care of the child prior to, or around the time of, their death. Contact should be made with other agencies who provided care to the child (e.g. CAMHS, speech and language therapy), both to inform them of the death and to gather any relevant information on the child and family. If child protection or safeguarding issues are raised, it may be necessary to take action to protect surviving siblings.

A decision will also be made at this time as to the appropriateness of a joint home visit (or a visit to the place where the child died) by a police officer and a senior health care professional. This would normally take place within the first 24–48 hours following the death. The health care professional who undertakes the home visit may be a paediatrician or a specialist nurse who is trained and experienced in unexpected death in childhood. The home visit provides an opportunity to gain additional information about the child, as well as an insight into parenting and environmental factors that may be helpful in determining the reasons for an unexpected child death. Viewing and discussing the sleeping arrangements for the child, including the sleeping surfaces, bedding and any co-sleeping can be particularly helpful. The joint visit also provides an opportunity to support parents and siblings and to provide information to them on other processes, such as the post-mortem examination.

The value of the visit being undertaken by a health professional who is able to benchmark home conditions and provision for the care of children based on extensive experience across diverse populations is self-evident, and is a role that is particularly suited to health visitors. Research undertaken with bereaved parents in areas in which there is an established tradition of joint visits has found that parents reported them to be helpful, rather than intrusive (Fleming *et al.* 2004).

Practice point

Chronic illness, disability and life-limiting conditions will account for a large proportion of deaths in childhood. These children and their families are likely to have had extensive engagement with a range of health care services. Professionals supporting the child and family will need to ensure appropriate support is in place, including end of life care plans, which may state where the child's body is to be cared for after their death (e.g. a cool room at a children's hospice). Although such deaths may be anticipated, they can also be unexpected and should be managed accordingly.

The local case discussion

The final phase of the rapid response comprises a local case discussion involving those who knew the child and family and those involved in investigating the death. This will take place once the post-mortem and ancillary investigations have been completed. The meeting is normally led by the designated paediatrician for unexpected child deaths (or their agreed deputy). Midwives, health visitors and/or school nurses are likely to be invited to contribute to this meeting. The main purpose is to:

- review the circumstances of the death;
- ensure the ongoing support of the family, including feedback of the outcomes of the local case discussion;
- highlight potential lessons to be learned;
- inform the coroner's inquest;
- provide a report of the local case discussion to the coroner and CDOP.

Case 2: Tegan – an unexpected death in infancy

Following a restless and difficult day, Tegan, who is 11 weeks old, falls asleep cuddled up with her mother Carys on the sofa. When Carys awakes at around 3 a.m. she realizes that Tegan is cold and pale. An ambulance is called and mother and baby are taken to the ED at the local general hospital. Sadly, Tegan is declared dead some 40 minutes later.

Sudden death in infancy

Sudden unexpected death in infancy (SUDI) is reported to be far less common than in the past and this has been related to changes made as a result of increased understanding of factors that may contribute to such deaths, especially those concerning safe sleeping practices (RCP/RCPCH 2004). Some SUDIs will be labelled as sudden infant death syndrome (SIDS), which is essentially a diagnosis of exclusion. There is, however, an association between SIDS and co-sleeping and recently updated NICE clinical guidelines on postnatal care advises that parents and carers are informed of the risks accordingly. As the guidance notes, co-sleeping may be intentional or unintentional and occur on a sofa, chair or bed. The risk is greater if mothers or their partners smoke, if they have recently consumed alcohol, in cases of parental drug use and if the infant was of a low birth weight and/or born preterm (NICE 2014c).

The leading non-SIDS causes have been noted to be infection, cardiovascular anomaly, child abuse and metabolic or genetic disorder (Loughrey et al. 2005). Parents will have 'mounting and reasonable' expectations that the cause of the death of their infant will be identified and it is thus important that any SUDI is thoroughly investigated (RCP/RCPCH 2004). Rapid response will assist with this.

Case 2 continued

Ceri, a named nurse for safeguarding children, has undertaken additional training to enable her to make a key contribution to the local rapid response process. Following the immediate care of the family and infant in the ED and a multi-agency strategy discussion, Ceri undertakes a joint home visit with a non-uniformed police officer from the local child abuse investigation unit.

At the home visit, Ceri is able to offer bereavement support to Tegan's family and make an assessment of the home conditions, in particular, the infant care and sleeping arrangements. She notes that the flat is very warm and that there is a smell of stale tobacco smoke. Ceri also gathers information from the health visitor who had undertaken an antenatal visit and new birth visit. Reports of the home visit are shared at the second strategy meeting at which a preliminary finding of cause of death from the post-mortem examination is reported as 'positional asphyxia'. No further significant information is raised at the final strategy meeting which meets to review the case and to consider ongoing support to the family, as well as issues that will be reported to the local CDOP.

The CDOP notes Tegan's death as part of its responsibility to undertake an overview of all deaths in the area. The panel also decides to review the case in more depth at a future meeting. This means that further information will be gathered from each agency so that factors in the child, family and environment, parenting capacity and service provision can be more fully discussed and recommendations made. Table 8.3 highlights the type of information that may be provided by the health visitor on the family and the child.

Learning from child death review processes

The case of Tegan demonstrates how child death review processes can be used to support bereavement care and learning to prevent future deaths. Nurses and midwives have a major role to play in contributing at a number of levels. Because there have been several SUDIs in the local authority area, the LSCB decide to launch a 'Safe Sleep' campaign based on the CDOP recommendations. This is led by a midwife and a police officer, with support from the local

Table 8.3 Information for a CDOP

Child	Family and environment
Normal delivery at 36 weeks' gestation	Few details known about father
Healthy small infant, birth weight 2.43 kg	Mother states not in a relationship
First child of young mother	Mother smoked 6–10 cigarettes per day during pregnancy, says to have reduced and smokes outside
Initially breast fed, but formula since 3 weeks of age	Drinks 1–2 units of alcohol daily (cider)
Slow to gain weight, last recorded weight 3.56 kg	Privately rented flat
Smiled at 7 weeks of age	Heating kept turned up due to tendency for dampness
Noted to have had a mild nappy rash at visit to child health clinic, otherwise has appeared well cared for	On benefits
Not yet had first immunization	Last worked as a retail assistant pre-pregnancy
	Own mother lives locally
	Few friends

Parenting capacity	Services provided
Enjoyed pregnancy and attended for all antenatal care	Shared care arrangements with maternity department and GP
Some support from own mother, but found role as single parent tiring	Assessed as low risk at new birth contact and invited to attend child health clinic at local children's centre
Warm and loving relationship with Tegan	Not seen by HV antenatally due to staff shortages caused by recruitment difficulties
SIDS prevention discussed (including safe sleep)	

CCG, NHS Trusts and police. Following the campaign there is a drop in the number of SUDIs reported locally and the campaign is shared more widely across the region. At any point before or during the rapid response or CDOP processes, concerns may arise as to the possibility of child maltreatment as a contributory factor in the death of a child or young person. In these instances, SCR processes will be instigated.

Summary

This chapter has considered statutory child death and SCR processes. Named and designated professionals play an important role. Designated nurses may be members of LSCB CDOPs and SCR committees. Named nurses (and specialist safeguarding nurses in their teams) may carry out the senior health care professional role as part of the rapid response. They will also support the SCR process by contributing written reports and/or supporting and debriefing front-line practitioners involved in these reviews. Nurses and midwives who provide care to children, young people and their families may find themselves contributing to SCRs or child death review processes.

The serious case review of Child HH, who died from DKA, provides a wealth of learning and improvement activity for health care organizations and professionals working with children, young people and their families. The unexpected death of Tegan, likewise, contributed to local activities to promote safe sleep in infancy. Enacting recommendations for practice improvement can thus be a positive force arising from rare, but sentinel, child deaths and child maltreatment tragedies.

Key points

- The prime purpose of an SCR is to learn lessons from serious child care incidents and child maltreatment deaths and to improve the safeguarding children practice of individuals and agencies.
- Contributing to an SCR can be a stressful experience and it is important that feedback and the opportunity to debrief are offered.
- Child death review processes provide opportunities to prevent future child deaths and to impact more widely on the health and well-being of children, young people and their families.
- Death rates of children are higher within families suffering the greatest socioeconomic difficulties.
- The child death review process provides an additional opportunity for inter-agency consideration of the possibility of maltreatment as a contributory factor.
- Recommendations for practice improvement can be a positive force arising from child maltreatment tragedies.

9
Messages for practice

Learning outcomes

This final chapter will help you to:

- Embed your learning about safeguarding and child protection in practice.
- Maximize your potential to make a difference to the outcomes of children, young people and their families.
- Promote the importance of the unique contribution of nurses, midwives and health visitors to the safeguarding and child protection processes.
- Practise with enhanced confidence.

Introduction

The second edition of this practical text has aimed to update and develop the safeguarding and child protection knowledge, skills, competence and unique contribution of the nursing, midwifery and health visiting workforce. The intention has been to reflect the full spectrum of safeguarding children work, from prevention and early intervention through to the contribution to child death and SCR, to give examples of different types of child maltreatment and to reflect the input of a range of nursing and midwifery practitioners in acute and community settings (see also Powell, in press). The basis for learning has been the case scenarios, in which the aim has been to highlight good practice. The text has been supported by reference to the evidence base – much of the policy, legislation and guidance is easily accessible via the internet and readers may like to develop their knowledge further through perusal of key texts.

This final chapter provides an opportunity to reinforce learning. However, it is also suggested that the best practice learning is experiential and readers are encouraged to seek opportunities to develop their knowledge, skills and competence. An approach can be made to safeguarding leads – i.e. named and designated professionals – who will be delighted to arrange shadowing activities and to share learning from local cases. I hope that together we can give birth to a new generation of nursing and midwifery safeguarding leads.

There follows a list of key learning points from the book as a whole, a safeguarding and child protection quiz for you to test your knowledge, and finally a checklist that will help you to consider the sources of support that you can access to improve your own safeguarding and child protection ractice.

Key learning points

- Safeguarding children applies to individuals from pre-birth to 18 years of age.
- Children's rights and child-centredness are essential to the delivery of safe, effective care and the achievement of best outcomes.
- Parents have the overriding responsibility to ensure that their children are safe; fathers, as well as mothers, need to be included in decision-making and care of their children.
- Child maltreatment is a major contemporary public health issue, but it is also open to a public health solution.
- Authoritative practice can help to ensure a timely and helpful response to children who may be in need of safeguarding and protection from harm.
- Nurses, midwives and health visitors have a range of opportunities to contribute to the prevention and early identification of child abuse and neglect.
- The FNP may confer a range of improved outcomes for the most vulnerable families including a reduction in child maltreatment.
- The EHA process provides a framework to assess strengths and needs within a family and to ensure timely support.
- Those providing contraception and sexual health services need to practise within the framework of legislation and guidance. This will include supporting children and young people's safety, as well as their health.
- Nurses and midwives who see children in the course of their practice should be familiar with child care and development and have a good understanding of indicators of possible child maltreatment.
- Health visitors and school nurses should be informed of all attendances at EDs/minor injuries units.
- A liaison health visitor/children's nurse can support information-sharing processes (two-way) between hospitals and community teams.
- Children attending for urgent care should have their child protection status checked.
- Children's social care and the police are the lead agencies for referral of child protection concerns; telephone referrals to children's social care should be followed up in writing within 48 hours.
- Clear, contemporaneous records of events and actions should be kept.

- In cases of suspected FII, a robust chronology detailing all contacts with health professionals should be drawn up.
- Support and advice on any aspect of safeguarding children can be obtained from named and designated professionals.
- An understanding of the needs of children and the features of good parenting is helpful in the prevention, early identification and response to emotional abuse.
- Assessments of children in need consider the child's developmental factors, family and environmental factors and parenting capacity.
- Sensitivity to race, culture and ethnicity is important, however, child abuse cannot be condoned for religious or cultural reasons.
- Child protection conferences should consider strengths and protective factors, as well as risks.
- Children and young people who are sexually abused experience difficulty in telling their story; victims are not always aware that what is happening to them is abusive.
- The effects of child sexual abuse are enduring and may be lifelong.
- Children who are disabled have a threefold risk of being abused, but are under-represented in safeguarding systems.
- Confidentiality in a patient–client relationship is *not* absolute; this should be explained to clients at the outset of any therapeutic relationship; in the case of Stewart, the 'public interest' would be *se*rved by reporting his online activity to the police.
- CSE is pernicious in its effects and raises some fundamental questions about the way in which children and young people (especially 'bad' children and young people) are viewed.
- Those individuals presenting with symptoms of CSE need to have the cause of their symptoms identified.
- Children and young people are groomed into CSE; at least initially many of them will genuinely believe that they are in a loving and consensual relationship.
- Children and young people are victims of CSE, not 'child prostitutes'. Perpetrators are committing criminal acts.
- Nurses, midwives and health visitors can escalate their concerns about poor practice through reference to organizational whistle-blowing policies.
- In cases of professional disagreement, LSCB escalation policies apply. Advice and support can be given by named nurses and their teams.
- Neglect is the most common reason for children and young people to have a child protection plan.
- An essential theme of neglect is 'omission' or 'absence of care'; the effects are cumulative.

- Neglect can lead to serious outcomes for children and young people, including fatality. It co-exists with other forms of abuse.
- When children do not attend health appointments this should be conceived as 'was not brought' rather than 'did not attend'.
- Professionals working with neglectful families need to ensure that they access high-quality supervision that will both support and challenge their thinking.
- The prime purpose of an SCR is to learn lessons from serious child care incidents and child maltreatment deaths and to improve the safeguarding children practice of individuals and agencies.
- Contributing to an SCR can be a stressful experience and it is important that feedback and the opportunity to debrief are offered.
- Child death review processes provide opportunities to prevent future child deaths and to impact more widely on the health and well-being of children, young people and their families.
- Death rates of children are higher within families suffering the greatest socioeconomic difficulties.
- The child death review process provides an additional opportunity for inter-agency consideration of the possibility of maltreatment as a contributory factor.
- Recommendations for practice improvement can be a positive force arising from child maltreatment tragedies.

Safeguarding and child protection quiz

1   Who are the lead statutory agencies for safeguarding children?
2   What are the seven golden rules of information-sharing?
3   What is positive parenting?
4   What are the three domains for assessment of children in need/an Early Help Assessment (EHA)?
5   What are the benefits of the Family Nurse Partnership (FNP) programme?
6   What is the most common sign of physical abuse?
7   Why is bruising in a non-mobile child of concern?
8   What features would lead you to suspect non-accidental thermal injury?
9   What is fabricated and induced illness (FII) and how may this present?
10   What is the timescale for following up a telephone referral to children's social care?

11 What is tier-two child and adolescent mental health services (CAMHS)?

12 What happens at a strategy discussion?

13 How may young people be groomed for sexual exploitation?

14 What is the most common category for children and young people made subject to a child protection plan?

15 What is another term for 'failure to thrive'?

16 What is the purpose of the core group?

17 How often should a child protection plan be reviewed and where does this happen?

18 What is the purpose of a chronology?

19 What is a genogram?

20 What are the benefits of clinical supervision in safeguarding children?

21 What are the steps of the rapid response to unexpected deaths in childhood?

22 What is the primary purpose of the child death overview panel (CDOP)?

23 What percentage of child deaths lead to a serious case review?

24 How can learning from serious case reviews improve practice?

Support for practice: are the following in place for you?

	Tick
I have access to my organization's safeguarding children policy and procedures, including those concerning children not brought to appointments and whistle-blowing	
I have access to my LSCB policy and procedures and I understand how to escalate concerns about a child	
I know how to contact my named and designated professionals	
I know how to contact my local children's social care department and the police, in and out of 'office hours'	
I know how to contact my LADO if I am concerned that a colleague poses a child protection risk to children in their care	
I have regular clinical/child protection supervision	
I update my safeguarding and child protection knowledge in accordance with mandatory training and the guidance provided by the RCPCH (2014)	

Conclusion

The importance of safeguarding and child protection being 'everyone's responsibility' has been promoted throughout this book. This includes all registrants
of the nursing and midwifery professions – i.e. nurses, midwives and specialist
community public health nurses (especially health visitors and school nurses)
who commission, manage or provide services to children, young people and
their families. At the time of writing, there are reported to be 680,000 nurses
and midwives on the professional register in the UK. Given the 'reach' of this
workforce into families and communities, there is much that can be achieved
by simply adhering to and learning from, the basics of good safeguarding children practice outlined in this book. The key to success is informed, authoritative practice that keeps a focus firmly on the child, a low threshold for concerns
and high expectations of parents and service delivery. Taking such a stance
provides us with the best opportunity to ensure that no more child protection
'scandals' bring shame and sorrow to families, communities, health professionals, the wider children's workforce and society as a whole. The children, young
people and families introduced throughout this book are, with the exception
of Child HH, not 'real', but their situations are very much so. Ultimately, I have
written this book to help nursing, midwifery and health visiting professionals
ensure that they are confident, competent and responsive in their safeguarding
and child protection practice.

A final note

Safeguarding and child protection work can be challenging. This is particularly the case for practitioners who may have their own histories of child maltreatment. If this book has raised specific concerns for you, or you know of
colleagues or adult clients who are seeking additional help to deal with unresolved issues, may I suggest that a good source of support is available from the
National Association for People Abused in Childhood (NAPAC). Their website is
as follows: http://napac.org.uk/ or they can be contacted free on 0808 801 0331.

Appendix

Safeguarding and child protection policy in England

Widely referred to as *Working Together*, the statutory guidance for England (HM Government 2015a) notes that safeguarding and child protection is 'everyone's responsibility'. This includes those who are providing services primarily for adults who may be parents or carers. The guidance outlines expectations that 'all agencies and professionals' will provide timely and proportionate help to families; be alert to potential indicators of maltreatment and the risks that abusers may pose to children; share and analyse information appropriately to inform assessments of harm; make a contribution to safeguarding and promoting the child's welfare; take part in reviews against specific plans and work cooperatively with parents (unless this would place the child at greater risk). Health bodies are named alongside other statutory agencies in having a duty under Section 11 of the Children Act 2004 to ensure that 'their functions are discharged with regard to the need to safeguard and promote the welfare of children' (p. 52). This applies to all those working in the health sector, whether they are working for NHS organizations or for services which are contracted out by the NHS to other providers, or provided independently. It is notable that provision for safeguarding and child protection is a key aspect of regulatory expectations and inspection.[1]

Safeguarding and child protection policy in Wales

The Welsh government takes the lead for policy for children and young people in Wales. It is supported by 'Children in Wales', an umbrella organization for organizations and individuals who work with children, young people and their families in Wales, who promote the development of the All Wales Child Protection Procedures[2] as part of their broader work to embed the UNCRC (1989). Wales also has a version of *Working Together* as the principality's statutory guidance (WAG 2007). This document outlines the roles and responsibilities of those working and volunteering with children, young people and their families in Wales. In 2016, a new legal obligation on public bodies to report any

---

[1]The CQC regulates health and social care provision and this includes review of arrangements for safeguarding children and young people. See http://www.cqc.org.uk/.
[2]http://www.awcpp.org.uk/home/wales-protocols/.

child or adult at risk of abuse or neglect will be introduced as part of the Social Services and Well-being (Wales) Act 2014. This new legislation will apply to local health boards and NHS Trusts in Wales.

Safeguarding and child protection policy in Scotland

In Scotland, child protection is the responsibility of the Scottish government. In conjunction with new legislation, the Children and Young People (Scotland) Act 2014, the government has updated its inter-agency child protection guidance (Scottish Government 2014), while also providing comprehensive bespoke guidance for health boards and professionals (Scottish Government 2013). As with the policy of other countries of the UK, there are explicit links to the UNCRC (1989). There are also specific links to Scotland's wider framework for children's safety and well-being known as *Getting it Right for Every Child* (GIRFEC).[3] Under the GIRFEC approach, each child has a named person from universal services who is responsible for assessment and who acts as a point of contact for the family and others supporting the child. Midwives, public health nurses/health visitors and family nurses (if involved) act as the named person until the child is of school age. Scottish guidance supports the importance of promoting the child protection role of health professionals whose primary client may be a parent, carer or another adult.

Safeguarding and child protection policy in Northern Ireland

In Northern Ireland, the responsibility for safeguarding and child protection rests with the Northern Ireland executive government, with support from the independent Safeguarding Board of Northern Ireland, which was established as a result of legislative changes in 2012. The key policy for safeguarding and child protection sits with the Department of Health, Social Services and Public Safety (DHSSPS 2003), with a wider 10-year strategy[4] for children supporting improvements in safeguarding alongside the implementation of the UNCRC (1989) in the country. The roles and expectations of health and social care boards, Trusts and individual professionals are set out in the policy.

[3]http://www.gov.scot/Topics/People/Young-People/gettingitright.
[4]http://www.delni.gov.uk/ten-year-strategy_1_.pdf.

References

ACMD (Advisory Council on the Misuse of Drugs) (2003) *Hidden Harm: Responding to the Needs of Children of Problem Drug Users*. London: Home Office/ACMD.

Action for Children (2014) *The Scandal that Never Breaks*. Watford: Action for Children.

All Party Parliamentary Group Conception to Age 2 – the first 1001 Days (2015) *Building Great Britons*, http://www.1001criticaldays.co.uk/buildinggreatbritonsreport. pdf (accessed 20 May 2015).

All Wales Child Protection Procedures Review Group (2008) *All Wales Child Protection Procedures*, http://www.awcpp.org.uk/wp-content/uploads/2014/03/All-Wales-Child-Protection-Procedures (accessed 12 May 2015).

Allnock, D. and Miller, P. (2013) *No One Noticed, No One Heard: A Study of Disclosures of Child Abuse*. London: NSPCC.

Ball, M., Barnes, J. and Meadows, P., (2012) *Issues Emerging From the First 10 Pilot Sites Implementing the Nurse-Family Partnership Home-visiting Programme in England*. London: DH.

Barlow, J. and Schrader-Macmillan, A. (2009) *Safeguarding Children from Emotional Abuse – What Works?* London: DfES.

Barnardo's Cymru (2013) *Sexual Exploitation Referral and Assessment Tool (SERAF)*. Wales: Barnardo's.

Barnes, J., Ball, M., Meadows, P., Belsky, J. and the FNP Implementation Research Team (2009) *Nurse–Family Partnership Programme Second Year Pilot Sites Implementation in England: The Infancy Period*. London: Institute for the Study of Children, Families and Social Issues, Birkbeck, University of London.

Bass, C. and Glaser, D. (2014) Early recognition and management of fabricated or induced illness in children, *Lancet* 383: 1412–21.

Berelowitz, S., Clifton, J., Firmin, C., Gulyurtlu, S. and Edwards, G. (2013) *'If Only Someone had Listened': Office of the Children's Commissioner's Inquiry into Child Sexual Exploitation in Gangs and Groups Final Report*. London: OCC.

Birmingham Safeguarding Children Board (2010) *Serious Case Review Under Chapter VIII 'Working Together to Safeguard Children' in Respect of the Death of a Child, Case Number 14*. Birmingham: Birmingham Safeguarding Children Board.

Brandon, M., Bailey, S., Belderson, P., *et al.* (2008) *Analysing Child Deaths and Serious Injuries through Abuse and Neglect: What Can We Learn? A Biennial Analysis of Serious Case Reviews 2003–2005*. London: DCSF.

Brandon, M., Bailey, S., Belderson, P., and Larsson, B. (2014a) The role of neglect in child fatality and serious injury, *Child Abuse Review* 23: 235–45.

Brandon, M., Glaser, D., Maguire, S., McCrory, E., Lushey, C., and Ward, H. (2014b) *Missed Opportunities: Indicators of Neglect – What is Ignored, Why, and What Can be Done?* London: Child Well-being Research Centre/Department for Education.

Brandon, M., Sidebotham, P., Bailey, S., Belderson, P., Hawley, C., Ellis, C. and Megson, M. (2012) *New Learning from Serious Case Reviews: A Two-year Report for 2009–2011*. London: DfE.

Bunn, A. (2013) *Signs of Safety® in England: An NSPCC Commissioned Report on the Signs of Safety Model in Child Protection*. London: NSPCC.

Burton, S. (2009) The oversight and review of cases in the light of changing circumstances and new information: how do people respond to new (and challenging) information? *Safeguarding Children Briefing 3*. London: Centre for Excellence in Outcomes for Children (C4EO).

Butchart, A., Harvey A.P. and Furniss T. (2006) *Preventing Child Maltreatment: A Guide to Taking Action and Generating Evidence*. Geneva: WHO and ISPCAN.

Cass, H. (2014) Child protection: a blend of art and science, *Archives of Disease in Childhood* 99: 101–2.

CEMACH (Confidential Enquiry into Maternal and Child Health) (2008) *Why Children Die*. London: CEMACH.

Child Exploitation and Online Protection Centre (CEOP) (2012) *A Picture of Abuse: A Thematic Assessment of the Risk of Contact Child Sexual Abuse Posed by those Who Possess Indecent Images of Children*. London: CEOP.

Cleaver, H., Nicholson, D., Tarr, S. and Cleaver, D. (2008) *Child Protection, Domestic Violence and Parental Substance Misuse: Family Experiences and Effective Practice*. London: DCSF.

Corby, B., Shemmings, D. and Wilkins, D. (2012) *Child Abuse: An Evidence Base for Confident Practice*, 4th edn. Maidenhead: Open University Press.

CQC (Care Quality Commission) (2009) *Safeguarding Children: A Review of the Arrangements in the NHS for Safeguarding Children*. London: CQC.

Daniel, B. (2015) Why have we made neglect so complicated? *Child Abuse Review* 24: 82–94.

Daniel, B., Taylor, J. and Scott, J., with Derbyshire, D. and Neilson, D. (2011) *Recognising and Helping the Neglected Child*. London: Jessica Kingsley.

Davies, C. and Ward, H. (2012) *Safeguarding Children Across Services: Messages from Research*. London: Jessica Kingsley.

Dean, E. (2014) The hidden toll of FGM, *Nursing Standard* 28(36): 20–2.

DCSF/DH (Department for Children, Schools and Families/Department of Health) (2009) *Getting Maternity Services Right for Pregnant Teenage Teenagers and Young Fathers*. London: DCSF.

De Laar, F. and Lagro-Jansson, T. (2009) Child protection: a Dutch GP's perspective, in J. Taylor and M. Themessl-Huber (eds) *Safeguarding Children in Primary Health Care*, pp. 39–48. London: Jessica Kingsley.

DfE (Department for Education) (2012) *What to Do if You Suspect a Child is Being Sexually Exploited: A Step By Step Guide For Frontline Practitioners*. London: DfE.

DfE (Department for Education) (2014a) *Statistical First Release: Characteristics of children in need 2013–2014*. London: DfE.

DfE (Department for Education) (2014b) *First Annual Report – National Panel of Independent Experts on Serious Case Reviews*. London: DfE.

DfE/DH (Department for Education, Department of Health (2014) *Special Educational Needs and Disability Code of Practice 0–25*. London: DfE.

DfES (Department for Education and Skills) (2004) *Every Child Matters: Change for Children*. London: DfES.

DH (Department of Health) (2009) *Improving Safety, Reducing Harm: Children, Young People and Domestic Violence. A Practical Toolkit for Front-line Professionals.* London: DH.

DH (Department of Health) (2011) *You're Welcome: Quality Criteria for Young People Friendly Health Services.* London: DH.

DH (Department of Health) (2012) *Health Visitor Implementation Plan 2011–2015.* London: DH.

DH (Department of Health) (2013) *A Framework for Sexual Health Improvement in England.* London: DH.

DH (Department of Health) (2014) *Developing Strong Relationships and Supporting Positive Sexual Health.* London: DH.

DH (Department of Health) (2015) *Female Genital Mutilation Risk and Safeguarding; Guidance for Professionals.* London: DH.

DH/DCSF (Department of Health, Department for Children, Schools and Families) (2009a) *Healthy Child Programme: Pregnancy and the First Five Years.* London: DH.

DH/DCSF (Department of Health, Department for Children, Schools and Families) (2009b) *Healthy Child Programme from 5–19 Years Old.* London: DH.

DH (Department of Health)/Health Working Group (2014) *Report on Child Sexual Exploitation: An Independent Group Chaired by the Department of Health Focusing on Improving the Outcomes for Children by Promoting Effective Engagement of Health Services and Staff.* London: DH.

DHSSPS (Department of Health, Social Services and Public Safety) (2003) *Co-operating to Safeguard Children.* Belfast: DHSSPS.

Dingwall, R., Eekalaar, J. and Murray, T. (1983) *The Protection of Children: State, Intervention and Family Life.* Oxford: Blackwell.

Easton, C., Morris, M. and Gee, G. (2010) *LARC2: Integrated Children's Services and the CAF Process.* Slough: NFER.

Eckenrode, J., Campa, M., Luckey, D. *et al.* (2010) Long-term effects of prenatal and infancy nurse home visitation on the life course of youths, *Archives Pediatric Adolescent Medicine* 164(1): 9–15.

Ferguson, H. (2012) Fathers, child abuse and child protection, *Child Abuse Review* 21: 231–36.

Ferguson, L. (2009) Proactive in protection: a public health approach to child protection, in J. Taylor and M. Themessl-Huber (eds) *Safeguarding Children in Primary Health Care.* London: Jessica Kingsley.

Fleming, P., Blair, P., Sidebotham, P. and Haylor, T. (2004) Investigating sudden unexpected deaths in infancy and childhood and caring for bereaved families: an integrated multi-agency approach, *British Medical Journal* 328: 331–4.

Fong, J. (2014) A critical analysis of the school nursing vision and call to action, *British Journal of School Nursing* 9(6): 287–5.

Fox, J. (2008) *A Contribution to the Evaluation of Recent Developments in the Investigation of Sudden Unexpected Deaths in Infancy.* Guildford: University of Surrey/National Policing Improvement Agency.

Gardner, R. (2008) *Developing an Effective Response to Emotional Harm and Neglect in Children.* Norwich: University of East Anglia and NSPCC.

Gaw, S. (2000) *What Works With Parents With Learning Disabilities?* Basildon: Barnardo's Publications.

Geib, A-J., Babu, K., Ewald, M. and Boyer, E. (2006) Adverse effects in children after unintentional buprenorphine exposure, *Pediatrics* 118: 1746–51.

Gilbert, R., Kemp, A., Thoburn, J. *et al.* (2008) Recognising and responding to child mal-treatment, *Lancet*, DOI:10.1016/S0140-6736(08)61707-9 (accessed 23 May 2015).

Gilbert, R. Widom, C.S., Brown, K., Fergusson, D., Webb, F. and Johnson, S. (2009) Burden and consequences of maltreatment in high income countries, *Lancet* 373: 68–81.

Golden, M., Samuels, M.P. and Southall, D.P. (2003) How to distinguish between neglect and deprivational abuse, *Archives of Disease in Childhood* 88: 105–7.

Gray, D. and Watt, P. (2013) *Giving Victims a Voice: Joint Report into Sexual Allegations Made Against Jimmy Savile.* London: Metropolitan Police Service/NSPCC.

Haringey Local Safeguarding Children Board (2009) *Serious Case Review: Child 'A' Published by the Department for Education on 26th October* 2010. London: DfE.

Herefordshire Safeguarding Children Board (2014) *Child HH: Overview Report.* Hertfordshire: HSCB.

HM Government (2008a) *Safeguarding Children in Whom Illness is Fabricated or Induced. Supplementary Guidance to Working Together to Safeguard Children.* London: DCSF.

HM Government (2008b) *Safeguarding Children Who May Have Been Trafficked.* London: DCSF.

HM Government (2009) *Safeguarding Children and Young People from Sexual Exploitation.* London: DCSF.

HM Government (2012) *The Government's Alcohol Strategy.* London: Home Office.

HM Government (2013) *Sexual Violence against Children and Vulnerable People: National Group Progress Report and Action Plan.* London: Home Office.

HM Government (2014) *Multi-agency Practice Guidelines: Female Genital Mutilation.* London: Home Office.

HM Government (2015a) *Working Together to Safeguard Children: A Guide to Inter-Agency Working to Safeguard and Promote the Welfare of Children.* London: DfE.

HM Government (2015b) *Information Sharing: Advice for Practitioners Providing Safeguarding Services to Children, Young People, Parents and Carers.* London: DfE.

HM Government (2015c) *What to Do if you are Worried a Child is Being Abused: Advice for Practitioners.* London: DfE.

Hogg, S. (2014) *All Babies Count: The Dad Project.* London: NSPCC.

Horvath, M.A.H., Davidson, J.C., Grove-Hills, J., Gekoski, A. and Choak, C. (2014) *'It's a Lonely Journey': A Rapid Evidence Assessment on Intra-familial Child Sexual Abuse.* London: Office of the Children's Commissioner.

House of Commons Education Committee (2012) *Children First: The Child Protection System in England.* London: Stationery Office.

House of Commons Home Affairs Committee (2013) *Child Sexual Exploitation and the Response to Localised Grooming.* London: Stationery Office.

Jay A. (2014) *Independent Inquiry into Child Sexual Exploitation in Rotherham 1997–2013.* Rotherham: Rotherham Metropolitan Borough Council.

Jenny, C. and Isaac, R. (2006) The relationship between child death and child maltreat-ment, *Archives of Disease in Childhood* 91: 265–9.

Jütte, S., Bentley, H., Miller, P. and Jetha, N. (2014) *How Safe are our Children?* London: NSPCC.

Laming, Lord (2003) *The Victoria Climbié Inquiry: Report of an Inquiry by Lord Laming,* Cm 5730. London: Stationery Office.

Laming, Lord (2009) *The Protection of Children in England: A Progress Report.* London: Stationery Office.

Lampard, K. (2014) *Independent Oversight of NHS and Department of Health Investigations into Matters Relating to Jimmy Savile.* London: DH.

Lombard N. and McMillan L. (eds) (2013) *Violence Against Women: Current Theory and Practice in Domestic Abuse, Sexual Violence and Exploitation.* London: Jessica Kingsley.

Loughrey, C., Preece, M. and Green, A. (2005) Sudden unexpected death in infancy (SUDI), *Journal of Clinical Pathology* 58: 20–1.

Lullaby Trust (2013) *Child Death Review: A Guide for Parents and Carers.* London: Lullaby Trust.

Morrison, T. (2009) The role of the scholar-facilitator in generating practice knowledge to inform and enhance the quality of relationship-based social work practice with children and families. Doctoral thesis, University of Huddersfield.

Munro, E. (2011) *The Munro Review of Child Protection Final Report: A Child-centred System.* London: Stationery Office.

Munro, E., Taylor, J. and Bradbury-Jones, C. (2014) Understanding the causal pathways to child maltreatment: implications for health and social care policy and practice, *Child Abuse Review* 23: 61–74.

Murray, M. and Osborne, C. (2009) *Safeguarding Disabled Children: Practice Guidance.* London: DCSF and Children's Society.

Myers, J. Berliner, L., Briere, J. *et al.* (2002) *The APSAC Handbook on Child Maltreatment,* 2nd edn. London: Sage.

National Commission of Inquiry into the Prevention of Child Abuse (1996) *Childhood Matters,* Vols I and II. London: Stationery Office.

Natsal-3 Sexual Attitudes and Lifestyles in Britain, http://www.natsal.ac.uk/ (accessed 20/05/15).

NCCWCH (National Collaborating Centre for Women's and Children's Health) (2009) *When to Suspect Child Maltreatment.* London: RCOG Press.

Nelson, S. (2009) Preparing for the special challenge of sexual abuse, in J. Taylor and M. Themessl-Huber (eds) *Safeguarding Children in Primary Health Care.* London: Jessica Kingsley.

NHS England (2015) *Serious Incident Framework: Supporting Learning to Prevent Recurrence.* London: NHS England.

NICE (National Institute for Health and Clinical Excellence) (2007) *Methadone and Buprenorphine for the Management of Opioid Dependence: NICE Technology Appraisal Guidance 114.* London: NICE.

NICE (National Institute for Health and Clinical Excellence) (2010) *Looked-after Children NICE Public Health Guidance 28* (modified October 2013) London: NICE.

NICE (National Institute for Health and Clinical Excellence) (2014a) *Domestic Violence and Abuse: How Health Services, Social Care and the Organisations they Work with can Respond Effectively: NICE Public Health Guidance 50.* London: NICE.

NICE (National Institute for Health and Clinical Excellence) (2014b) *Health Visiting: NICE Local Government Briefings lgb22.* London: NICE.

NICE (National Institute for Health and Clinical Excellence) (2014c) *Post-natal Care: Clinical Guidance 37 (modified February 2015).* London: NICE.

NMC (Nursing and Midwifery Council) (2015) *The Code: Professional Standards of Practice and Behaviour for Nurses and Midwives.* London: NMC.

NSPCC (2013) *Learning from Serious Case Reviews around Childhood Sexual Exploitation,* http://www.nspcc.org.uk/preventing-abuse/child-protection-system/case-reviews/learning/child-sexual-exploitation/ (accessed 26 May 2015).

NSPCC (2014) *Child Killings in England and Wales: Explaining the Statistics*, http:// www.nspcc.org.uk/globalassets/documents/information-service/factsheet-child-killings-england-wales-homicide-statistics.pdf (accessed 21 May 2015).

NSPCC (2015) *Health: Learning from Case Reviews: Summary of Risk Factors and Learning for Improved Practice for the Health Sector (Paediatrics and Accident & Emergency)*, http://www.nspcc.org.uk/preventing-abuse/child-protection-system/ case-reviews/learning/health/ (accessed 27 May 2015).

Office of the First Minister and Deputy First Minister Northern Ireland (2006) *Our Children and Young People – Our Pledge: A Ten Year Strategy for Children and Young People in Northern Ireland 2006–2016*. Belfast: OFMDFM.

Ofsted (2012) *Protecting Disabled Children: Thematic Inspection*. London: Ofsted.

Ofsted (2014) *In the Child's Time: Professional Responses to Neglect*. London: Ofsted.

Olds, D.L., Eckenrode, J., Henderson, C.R. *et al.* (1997) Long-term effects of home visitation on maternal life course and child abuse and neglect, *Journal of the American Medical Association* 278(8): 637–43.

Olds, D.L., Henderson, C.R. and Kitzman, J. (1994) Does prenatal and infancy nurse home visitation have enduring effects on qualities of parental caregiving and child health at 25 to 50 months of life? *Pediatrics* 93: 1, 89–98.

Oxfordshire Safeguarding Children Board (2015) *Serious Case Review into Child Sexual Exploitation in Oxfordshire: From the Experiences of Children A, B, C, D, E, and F*. Oxford: Oxfordshire Safeguarding Children Board.

Pearce, J. (2013) 'What's going on' to safeguard children and young people from child sexual exploitation: a review of local safeguarding children boards' work to protect children from sexual exploitation, *Child Abuse Review* 23(3): 159–70.

Polnay, J., Polnay, L., Lynch, M. and Shabde, N. (eds) (2007) *A Child Protection Reader*. London: RCPCH.

Powell, C. (2007) *Safeguarding Children and Young People: A Guide for Nurses and Midwives*. Maidenhead: Open University Press.

Powell, C. (in press) Safeguarding and child protection: the important contribution of the wider nursing and midwifery workforce, in J. Appleton and S. Peckover (eds) *Child Protection, Public Health and Nursing*. Edinburgh: Dunedin Academic Press.

Powell, C. and Appleton, J. (2012) Children and young people's missed health care appointments: Reconceptualising 'did not attend' to 'was not brought' – a review of the evidence for practice, *Journal of Research in Nursing* 17(2): 181–92.

Princess Royal Trust for Carers/Children's Society (2010) *Supporting Young Carers: A Resource for Schools*. London: Princess Royal Trust for Carers.

Radford, L., Corral, S., Bradley, C., Fisher, H., Bassett, C., Howat, N. and Collishaw, S. (2011) *Child Abuse and Neglect in the UK Today*. London: NSPCC.

RCM/RCN/RCOG/Equality Now/UNITE (2013) *Tackling FGM in the UK: Intercollegiate Recommendations for Identifying, Recording, and Reporting*. London: Royal College of Midwives.

RCN/RCPCH (Royal College of Nursing, Royal College of Paediatrics and Child Health) (2015) *Looked After Children: Knowledge, Skills and Competence of Health Care Staff – Intercollegiate Role Framework*. London: RCPCH.

RCP/RCPCH (Royal College of Pathologists, Royal College of Paediatrics and Child Health) (2004) *Sudden Unexpected Death in Infancy: A Multi-Agency Protocol for Care and Investigation. The Report of a Working Group Convened by the*

Royal College of Pathologists, Royal College of Paediatrics and Child Health (The Kennedy Report). London: Royal College of Pathologists, Royal College of Paediatrics and Child Health.

RCPCH (Royal College of Paediatrics and Child Health) (2009) *Fabricated or Induced Illness by Carers (FII): A Practical Guide for Paediatricians*. London: RCPCH.

RCPCH (Royal College of Paediatrics and Child Health) (2012) *Standards for the Care of Children and Young People in Emergency Care Settings: Developed by the Intercollegiate Committee for Standards for Children and Young People in Emergency Care Settings*. London: RCPCH.

RCPCH (Royal College of Paediatrics and Child Health) (2014) *Safeguarding Children and Young People: Roles and Competences for Health Care Staff (Intercollegiate Guidance Third Edition)*. London: RCPCH.

Reder, P., Duncan, S. and Gray, M. (1993) *Beyond Blame: Child Abuse Tragedies Revisited*. London: Routledge.

Robert, K. and Harris, J. (2002) *Disabled People in Refugee and Asylum Seeking Communities*. Bristol: Policy Press.

Rochdale Borough Safeguarding Children Board (2012) *Child Sexual Exploitation Themed Review*. Rochdale: RBSCB.

Roe, M.F., Appleton, J.V. and Powell, C. (2015) Why was this child not brought? *Archives of Disease in Childhood* 100: 511–12.

Royal College of Physicians (2010) *Passive Smoking and Children*. London: RCP.

Royal College of Psychiatrists (2012) *Behavioural Problems and Conduct Disorder: Factsheet*. London: RCP.

Royal College of Radiologists/RCPCH (2008) *Standards for Radiological Investigations in Cases of Suspected Non-accidental Injury*. London: RCPCH.

SCIE (Social Care Institute for Excellence) (2005) *Research Briefing 9: Preventing Teenage Pregnancy in Looked After Children*, http://www.scie.org.uk/publications/briefings/briefing09/index.asp (accessed 19 May 2015).

Scottish Government (2013) *Child Protection: Guidance for Health Professionals*. Edinburgh: Scottish Government.

Scottish Government (2014) *National Guidance for Child Protection in Scotland*. Edinburgh: Scottish Government.

Sharma, A., and Cockerill, H. (2014) *Mary Sheridan's From Birth to Five Years: Children's Developmental Progress*. Abingdon: Taylor & Francis.

Shemmings, D. and Shemmings, Y. (2011) *Understanding Disorganized Attachment: Theory and Practice for Working with Children and Adults*. London: Jessica Kingsley.

Sidebotham, P. (2015) The challenge and complexities of physical abuse, *Child Abuse Review* 24: 1–5.

Sidebotham, P., Atkins, B. and Hutton, J. (2012) Changes in rates of violent child deaths in England and Wales between 1974 and 2008: an analysis of national mortality data, *Archives of Disease in Childhood* 97(3): 193–9.

Sidebotham, P., Brandon, M, Powell, C. *et al.* (2010) *Learning from Serious Case Reviews: Report of a Research Study on the Methods of Learning Lessons Nationally from Serious Case Reviews*. London: DfE.

Sidebotham, P., Fox, J., Horwath, J. and Powell, C. (2011) Developing effective child death review: a study of 'early starter' child death overview panels in England, *Injury Prevention* 17: i55–63.

Sidebotham, P., Fox, J., Horwath, J., Powell, C. and Perwez, S. (2008) *Preventing Childhood Deaths: A Study of 'Early Starter' Child Death Overview Panels in England*. London: DCSF.

Srivastava, O.P. and Polnay, L. (1997) Field trial of graded care profile (GCP) scale: a new measure of care, *Archives of Disease in Childhood* 76: 337–40.

Stanley, N. (2011) *Children Experiencing Domestic Violence: A Research Review*. Dartington: Research in Practice.

Stein, M., Rees, G., Hicks, L. and Gorin, S. (2009) *Neglected Adolescents: A Review of the Research and the Preparation of Guidance for Multi-Disciplinary Teams and a Guide for Young People*. London: DCSF.

Stratheam, L., Mamun, A., Najman, J. and O'Callaghan, M. (2009) Does breastfeeding protect against substantiated child abuse and neglect? A 15-year cohort study, *Pediatrics* 123: 483–93.

Taylor, J., Lauder, W., Moy, M. and Corlett, J. (2009) Practitioner assessments of 'good enough' parenting: factorial survey, *Journal of Clinical Nursing* 18: 11–9.

Taylor, J., Spencer, N. and Baldwin, N. (2000) Social, economic and political contexts of parenting, *Archives of Disease in Childhood* 82: 113–20.

Tuck, V. (2013) Resistant parents and child protection: knowledge base, pointers for practice and implications for policy, *Child Abuse Review* 22(5): 19.

UNICEF (2014) *Hidden in Plain Sight: A Statistical Analysis of Violence Against Children*. New York: UNICEF.

Vincent, S. (2009) *Child Death and Serious Case Review Processes in the UK*. Edinburgh: University of Edinburgh/NSPCC.

WAG (Welsh Assembly Government) (2007) *Safeguarding Children: Working Together Under the Children Act 2004*. Cardiff: WAG.

WCPSRG (Welsh Child Protection Systematic Review Group) (2014) *Distinguishing Intentional and Non-intentional Scalds in Children*, http://www.core-info.cardiff. ac.uk/reviews/burns/scalds-key-messages (accessed 21 May 2015).

WCPSRG/NSPCC (Welsh Child Protection Systematic Review Group, National Society for the Prevention of Cruelty to Children) (2012) *Core-Info: Bruises on Children*. Cardiff: University of Cardiff.

WHO (World Health Organization) (2006) *Preventing Child Maltreatment: A Guide to Taking Action and Generating Evidence*. Geneva: WHO and International Society for Prevention of Child Abuse and Neglect.

Wolfe, I., Macfarlane, A., Donkin, A., Marmot, M. and Viner, R. (2014) *Why Children Die: Death in Infants, Children, and Young People in the UK*. London: Royal College of Paediatrics and Child Health and National Children's Bureau.

Wright, C.M. (2005) What is weight faltering (failure to thrive) and when does it become a child protection issue? in J. Taylor and B. Daniel (eds) *Child Neglect: Practical Issues for Health and Social Care*. London: Jessica Kingsley.

Index

Locators shown in italics refer to figures and tables.